YOUR
CANNABIS
EXPERIENCE

YOUR CANNABIS EXPERIENCE

A BEGINNER'S GUIDE TO BUYING, GROWING, COOKING, AND HEALING WITH CANNABIS

SANDRA HINCHLIFFE

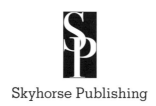

Skyhorse Publishing

Skyhorse Publishing books may be purchased in bulk at special discounts for sales promotion, corporate gifts, fund-raising, or educational purposes. Special editions can also be created to specifications. For details, contact the Special Sales Department, Skyhorse Publishing, 307 West 36th Street, 11th Floor, New York, NY 10018 or info@skyhorsepublishing.com.

Skyhorse® and Skyhorse Publishing® are registered trademarks of Skyhorse Publishing, Inc.®, a Delaware corporation.

Visit our website at www.skyhorsepublishing.com.

10 9 8 7 6 5 4 3 2 1

Library of Congress Cataloging-in-Publication Data is available on file.

Cover design by David Ter-Avanesyan
Cover photo credit by Sandra Hinchliffe

Print ISBN: 978-1-5107-5511-6
Ebook ISBN: 978-1-5107-5512-3

Printed in China

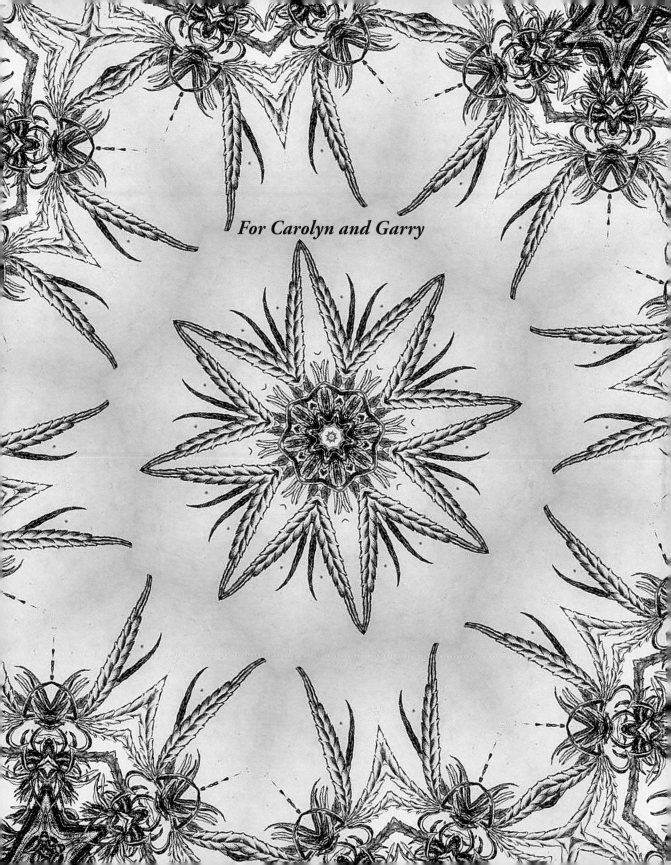

For Carolyn and Garry

CONTENTS

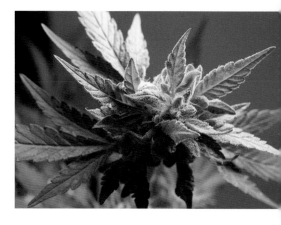

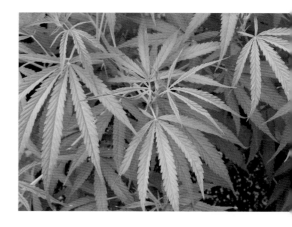

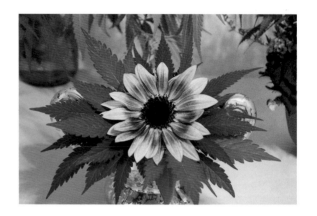

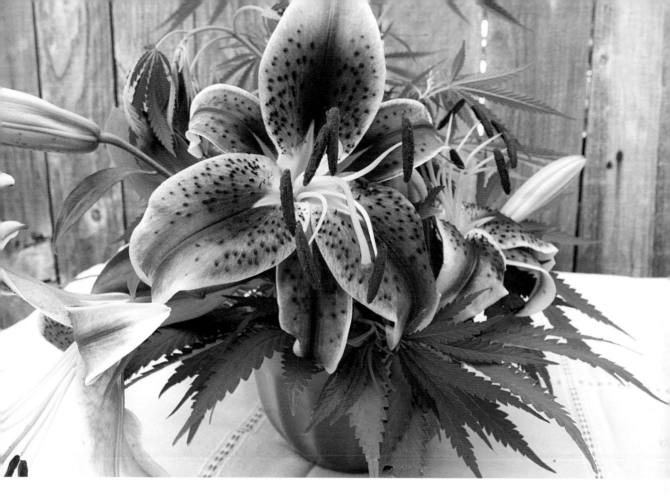

PREFACE

This book is intended for readers eighteen and older, and cannabis use only for those twenty-one and older and in locations where cannabis is legal. Please consult with an attorney if you have questions about the legality of cannabis in your area.

    Always consult with your private doctor if you have any questions about whether or not cannabis is right for you and appropriate to use along with other medications.

    This book is not intended to cure, treat, or diagnose any disease or condition.

    Never drive or operate dangerous machinery under the influence of any substance, even natural plant substances like cannabis.

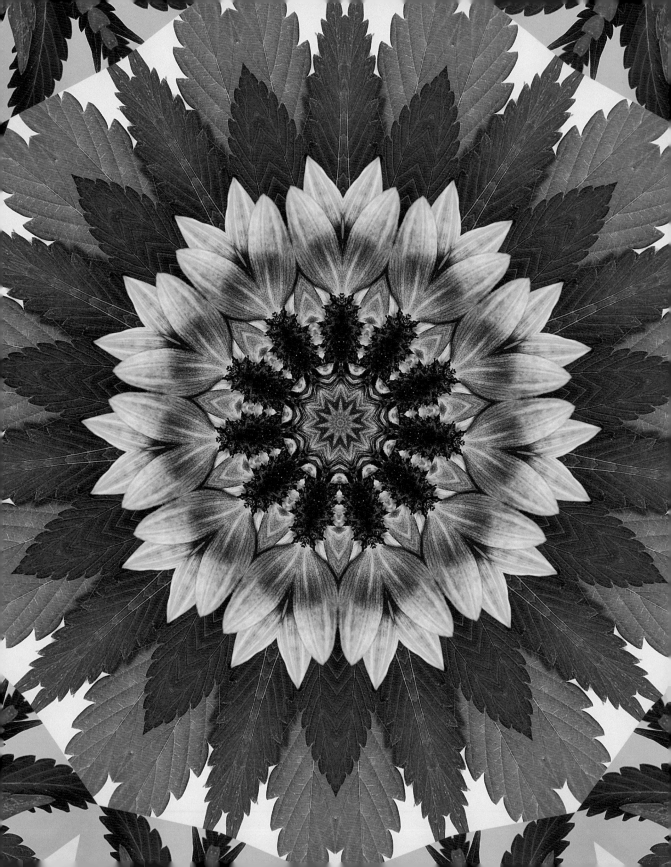

INTRODUCTION TO THE FABULOUS FLOWER LIFE

In fall 2012, I began production for a book about my niche in cannabis herbalism—cannabis topical and topical-transdermal formulations, such as cannabis-infused salves, lotions, and baths. I have been publishing cannabis-infused topical-transdermal recipes for other home herbalists on my website, posyandkettle.com, since 2009. My interest in this herbal niche, my frequent personal use and sharing of "cannabis spa" with my inner circle, and my experience as a home herbalist for more than twenty years led to the development of a portfolio of cannabis spa recipes and techniques that would eventually be published in my book. This book, *The Cannabis Spa at Home*, was my first book, but it also has the honor of being the first modern book to be published about cannabis-infused spa and topical-transdermal formulations.

I took a break while working on my first book one fall evening in 2012 to grab some takeout from my favorite restaurant. I overestimated my wellness that evening and ended up taking a (predictable) fall in the parking lot that would send me to the emergency room that night. Complicating and increasing the pain and swelling from the fall I had just taken was the fact that I was, at that time, still under the care of a rheumatologist and undergoing immunotherapy for a rare and very serious autoimmune disease that threatened my eyes and the functioning of my other organs and left my body in agony with pain.

That evening, I arrived at the emergency room and passed through triage rather quickly. I was given a bed, and my husband and I would be waiting there for some time until the radiology department was ready for my now severely swollen foot and ankle. As I was waiting, the bed next to mine was being prepared for another patient who was brought in by an ambulance. An eighty-three-year-old elderly woman who was in an extreme state of dysphoria, hallucinating, and gripping her chest in pain, had just arrived on a gurney accompanied by her family.

Because the beds are so close in the emergency room, with only a curtain to separate them, I could hear all of the conversations taking place in the bed next to mine. I listened as the family told the doctors that their grandmother had eaten 100 milligrams of THC in the form of a single cookie that was sold to her by a legal medical cannabis dispensary.

In California, in 2012, in order to purchase cannabis products from a legal medical cannabis dispensary, this grandmother would have had a medical recommendation document from a licensed physician. According to her family, she independently sought out a medical cannabis recommendation for arthritis because she was consuming a significant amount of prescription opioid medications. She wanted to stop taking these medications on a daily basis. The family also felt that this was a step in the right direction, since their grandmother was not happy with the side effects of taking prescription opioids every day. They seemed both baffled and frightened that this had happened to their grandmother and were concerned that perhaps there was something else in that cookie that was not medical marijuana due to the reaction she was now having.

After the physician ordered blood work to determine the substance she had ingested, which turned out to be THC, she was given IV medications and put on a heart monitor. The doctor explained to the family that they were very concerned about her high blood pressure reading and the possibility of heart attack and stroke. The psychoactive effects of the amount of THC she ingested had caused her to experience severe anxiety and an acute psychotic episode, and this was the reason for the high blood pressure. The doctor also reassured the family that she would probably be fine in a few hours, but that they would keep her there until they were sure that she had sufficiently come down from the "high" and her blood pressure and mental condition were stable again, and that the IV medications would facilitate this.

How did this happen? How did the California medical cannabis system fail her? Or did it? In my head, I noted where I believed the failure had happened in the new century of legalization: missed educational opportunities, number one. But also, dispensaries and manufacturers. The untrained dispensary staff who either didn't care or didn't understand that giving an elderly woman, a first-time cannabis consumer, a cannabis cookie containing 100 milligrams of THC and expecting her to remember all of the steps to divide it into 20 or more pieces before ingesting one small piece was wildly inappropriate and dangerous.

Of course, for the "reefer madness" prohibitionist, this grandmother is a perfect example of why cannabis should be illegal instead of being a perfect example of missed educational opportunities. No educational opportunities are necessary if cannabis were made illegal once again! After all, the medical cannabis advocates were wrong about the harmlessness of cannabis because people have had heart attacks due to psychotic episodes induced by the consumption of large amounts of THC! And they would be on point with this part of their argument because there are, in fact, numerous case reports in legitimate medical journals documenting the uptick of cardiac-related emergency room visits,[1] namely for edible THC cannabis products. For example:

> *The case report describes a 70-year-old man with stable coronary artery disease, taking the appropriate cardiac medications, who ate most of a lollipop that was infused with 90 mg of THC (delta-9-tetrahydrocannabinol) to relieve pain and aid sleep, which caused him to have a potentially-serious heart attack. . . . The patient's cardiac event was likely triggered by unexpected strain on his body from anxiety and fearful hallucinations caused by the unusually large amount of THC he ingested. His sympathetic nervous system was stimulated, causing increased cardiac output with tachycardia, hypertension, and catecholamine (stress hormone) release. After the psychotropic effects of the drug wore off, and his hallucinations ended, his chest pain stopped.*
>
> *A number of prior case reports, as well as epidemiological studies, have described the association between cannabis use and acute cardiovascular (CV) adverse events, including myocardial infarction, stroke, arrhythmias, and sudden death.*

However, the physician also notes the benefits of cannabis in this same article:

> *Marijuana can be a useful tool for many patients, especially for pain and nausea relief. At the same time, like all other medications, it does carry risk and side effects. In a recent case, inappropriate dosing and oral consumption of marijuana by an older patient with stable cardiovascular disease resulted in distress that caused a cardiac event and subsequent reduced cardiac function.*[2]

---

1   Kerwin McCrimmon, Katie. "Marijuana-related ER visits rising dramatically, edibles sparking particular concerns." *UCHealth.org.* https://www.uchealth.org/today/marijuana-related-er-visits-rising-dramatically -edibles-spraking-particular-concerns/

2   Leahy, Eileen. "Potent marijuana edibles can pose a major unrecognized risk to patients with cardiovascular disease." *Canadian Journal of Cardiology*, 2019. *EurekAlert*, https://www.eurekalert.org/news-releases /778750.

But the data doesn't bear out tales of reckless abandon in regards to these incidents as the prohibitionists would have us believe. The data, in most of these case reports, bears witness to the lingering vestiges of prohibition stigma—the dearth of cannabis education at a societal level. We've all received an education about the appropriate use of alcohol and prescription drugs beginning in childhood. But very few of us have received a comparable education about cannabis, and about using cannabis appropriately, due to the stigma that comes with prohibition.

As I was waiting for my X-ray, I continued to dwell on how this frightening and potentially dangerous situation did not have to happen to the grandmother in the bed next to me. I silently promised her that I would write a book just for her and her family. That in the future, after I had more experience with every aspect of cannabis, including growing cannabis, I would write a guide to a beneficial, safe, and enjoyable experience for everyone who wants to try cannabis for the first time, and for those who are revisiting cannabis for the first time in a long time.

This is that book.

This book is for every novice: young adults, senior citizens, and everyone in between, and for anyone who hasn't touched cannabis since college and now finds themselves living in a state or country that has recently legalized cannabis. And this book is for people who have had less than satisfying or uncomfortable experiences with cannabis, too.

I've been writing books featuring both nonpsychoactive and euphoric cannabis recipes and techniques for the past decade, and I want you to know that almost everyone can have a great experience with cannabis! Whether that is enjoying a nonpsychoactive experience with fan leaves as leafy green vegetables, topicals and spa, CBD, or a mindfully euphoric experience with flower vaping and a cookie. There are so many ways to experience the cannabis plant, and that's what I like to call the fabulous flower life!

The experience of the fabulous flower life embraces both the awe and reverence that this plant creates in its most ardent connoisseurs, as well as the respect and boundaries of temperate mindfulness. Cannabis is a beautiful and diverse plant with some of the most complex chemistry of any plant in existence. It deserves both reverence and respect. It is my hope that my canna-epicurean philosophy will resonate with you as you read this book.

—Sandra Hinchliffe

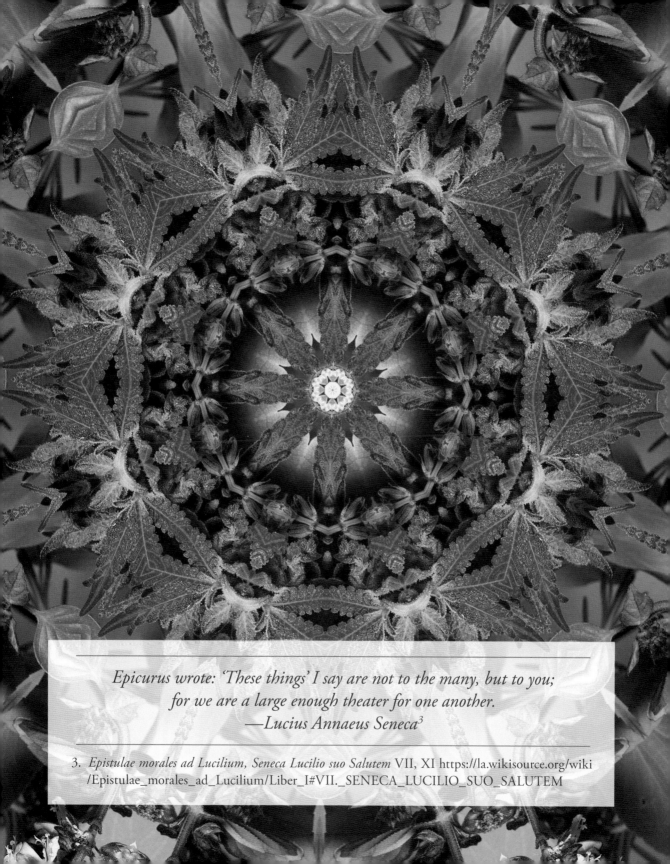

Epicurus wrote: 'These things' I say are not to the many, but to you;
for we are a large enough theater for one another.
—*Lucius Annaeus Seneca*[3]

3. *Epistulae morales ad Lucilium, Seneca Lucilio suo Salutem* VII, XI https://la.wikisource.org/wiki
/Epistulae_morales_ad_Lucilium/Liber_I#VII._SENECA_LUCILIO_SUO_SALUTEM

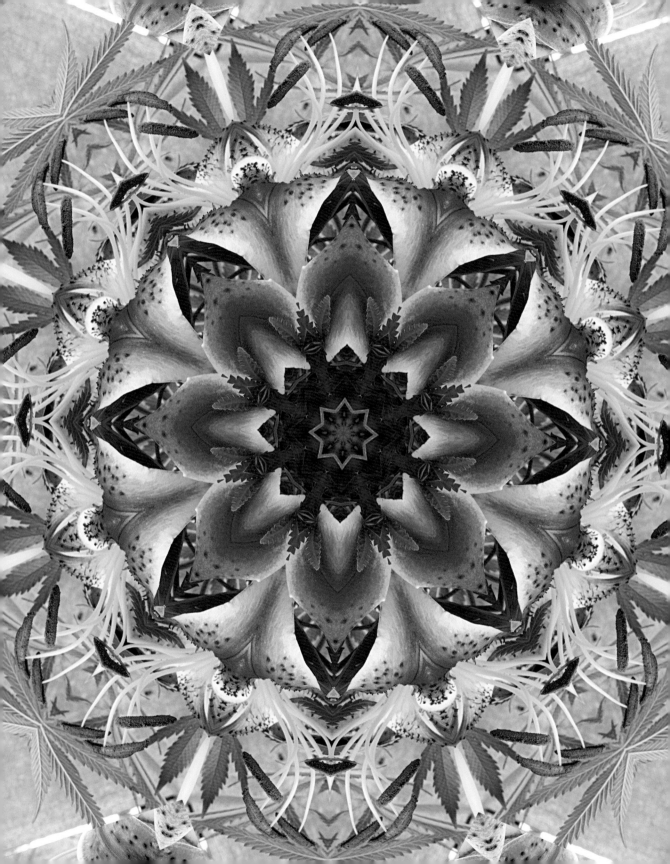

CHAPTER ONE

CANNABIS YESTERDAY, TODAY, AND FOREVER

Cannabis sativa L. has an ancient history and complex biology. You don't need a PhD to use cannabis, but beneficial, enjoyable, and safe experiences with cannabis begin with a few small servings of the history and science behind this plant.

Cannabis Evolution and the Modern Era: Cannabis Then and Now

We begin our journey with the cannabis plant around 19 million years ago somewhere on the Tibetan Plateau, where what is thought to be the oldest sample of cannabis pollen was found. But the cannabis plant had a much earlier beginning 10 million years prior when it diverged from its closest relative *Humulus lupulus,* hops.[1] Yes, the same hops used to make beer is the closest living relative of the cannabis plant! Both plants are dioecious (have both male and female flowers, usually on separate plants), and both plants produce a bitter, sticky resin—cannabis making phytocannabinoid and aromatic compounds, and hops making lupulin and aromatic compounds. Although I haven't been able to find any scientific literature on what exactly the characteristics were of the common ancestor, I've often wondered if the oldest common ancestor of both plants that lived 30 million years

An illustration depicting the female and male cannabis plant, as seen in *The Universal Herbal; or, Botanical, Medical, and Agricultural Dictionary*, by Thomas Greene, 1823. This book contains mostly plant identification illustrations that would have been useful in medicine or the medical agriculture of the era.

1 McPartland, J. M., W. Hegman, and T. Long. "Cannabis in Asia: its center of origin and early cultivation, based on a synthesis of subfossil pollen and archaeobotanical studies." *Veget Hist Archaeobot* 28, 691–702 (2019). https://doi.org/10.1007/s00334-019-00731-8

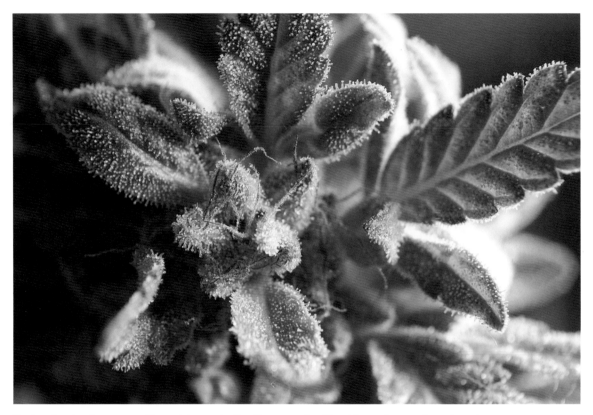

Resin glands of a mature *Cannabis* ssp. *indica* flower, unfertilized by pollen and ready to harvest.

ago produced a unique resinous compound that had the qualities of both phytocannabinoids and lupulin along with the aromatic compounds that they have in common today.

The human experience with cannabis in China, India, and the Middle and Near East begins with a subspecies of *Cannabis sativa L.* that has been identified in both historical and modern botanical and anthropology literature as *Cannabis* ssp. *indica*. This species of cannabis is most commonly associated with the thick production of medicinal and narcotic phytocannabinoid resins and known for its medicinal, spiritual, and euphoric uses. This plant is sometimes called Indian hemp. Herodotus wrote that the ancient Scythians cultivated the narcotic hemp and burned the seed heads over a fire to create what is known today as a "hot box"[2] of vapor for the purposes of euphoric ecstasy.

---

2 *Hotboxing* is a method of burning or vaporizing a large amount of cannabis in an open container in order to fill a small closed space with the smoke or vapor for the purposes of medicine and pleasure.

"In those remote times, the hemp and the poppy were not unknown; and there is reason for believing that in Egypt the former was used as a potion for soothing and dispelling care. Herodotus informs us that the Scythians cultivated hemp, and converted it into linen cloth, resembling that made from flax;" and he adds also, that "when, therefore, the Scythians have taken some seed of this hemp, they creep under the cloths, and then put the seed on the red hot stones; but this being put on smokes, and produces such a steam, that no Grecian vapour-bath would surpass it. The Scythians, transported with the vapour, shout aloud."* The same author also states that the Massagetse, dwelling on an island of the Araxes, have discovered "trees that produce fruit of a peculiar kind, which the inhabitants, when they meet together in companies, and have lit a fire, throw on the fire as they sit round in a circle; and that by inhaling the fumes of the burning fruit that has been thrown on, they become intoxicated by the odour, just as the Greeks do by wine, and that the more fruit is thrown on, the more intoxicated they become, until they rise up to dance, and betake themselves to singing."[3]

The use of cannabis in the Persian and Middle East was so common that it is mentioned often by scholars who have written about the botanical history of these regions. And these historical texts place cannabis in the regions associated with the Jewish Torah, Christian Bible, and Islamic Quran. The widespread use of cannabis among the cultures of this region of the world has been so well documented that it's not at all an unusual or edge-case interpretation to include cannabis as one of the many herbs that appear in both canonical and noncanonical scriptures.[4]

"Indian hemp has been long known in India, Persia, and other Eastern countries as a medicinal and intoxicating agent, but was little known to Europeans until it was brought prominently into notice by Dr O'Shaughnessy of Calcutta, in the year 1839. [On Indian Hemp, &c.; Calcutta, 1839.]"[5]

---

3 Cooke, M. C. *The Seven Sisters of Sleep: Popular History of the Seven Prevailing Narcotics of the World,* 10–11, 1860.
4 Thompson, R. Campbell. *The Assyrian Herbal,* p. 54, 64, 101, 1924. Boyce, Sidney Smith. *Hemp (Cannabis sativa): A Practical Treatise on the Culture of Hemp for Seed and Fiber, with a Sketch of the History and Nature of the Hemp Plant,* 4, 1900.
5 Christison, Alexander. *On the Natural History, Action, and Uses of Indian Hemp,* 3, 1851.

In the creation story shared among all the Abrahamic faiths, a gift from God:

Genesis 1:29 "And God said, behold I have given you every herb bearing seed, which is upon the face of all the earth, and every tree, which is the fruit of the tree yielding seed; to you it shall be for meat."

Sula Benet, a Polish anthropologist specializing in Judaism, has offered a compelling opinion based on the evidence of the widespread use of cannabis in this region; cannabis was a key ingredient in the anointing oil of the Old Testament priesthood,[6]

Exodus 30:22–25 Moreover the LORD spoke unto Moses, saying: 'Take thou also unto thee the chief spices, of flowing myrrh five hundred shekels, and of sweet cinnamon half so much, even two hundred and fifty, and of fragrant cane (kanehbos/kaneh-bosem) two hundred and fifty, and of cassia five hundred, after the shekel of the sanctuary, and of olive oil a hin. And thou shalt make it a holy anointing oil, a perfume compounded after the art of the perfumer; it shall be a holy anointing oil.

The King James and some other translations (but not all!) of the Bible translated the original Hebrew kaneh bosem קנה בשם as another herb, sweet calamus, which is a plant that contains toxins that are both cancerous and have insecticidal properties.[7] Sula Benet and other Jewish scholars have disagreed with this translation. The sweet cane or fragrant cane of the Old Testament was actually cannabis. The latter translation actually makes more sense in light of the use of this anointing oil, which contained a significant concentration of kaneh-bos/kaneh bosem, as it was poured over the head in priestly rituals.

---

6   Benet, Sula, "Early Diffusion and Folk Uses of Hemp." *Cannabis and Culture*, Rubin, Vera & Comitas, Lambros, (eds.) 1975. 39-49. https://web.archive.org/web/20210814165507/https://www.xn--4dbcyzi5a .com/wp-content/PDF/EARLY-DIFFUSION-AND-FOLK-USES-OF-HEMP-SULA-BENET.pdf
7   *"Acorus calamus."* Wikipedia.org, https://en.wikipedia.org/wiki/Acorus_calamus

In the Living Torah, a widely used English translation of the Torah, Orthodox Rabbi Aryeh Kaplan explains the possibility of several plants identified as "fragrant cane" and cites cannabis as one of these: "On the basis of cognate pronunciation and Septuagint readings, some identify keneh bosem with the English and Greek cannabis, the hemp plant." Rabbi Kaplan goes further to explain how this prescribed anointing ointment was to be made as a "blended compound" that involved one of two methods: cooking herbs with oil and water or cooking all of the herbs in oil. "The anointing oil was made by soaking the aromatic substances in water until the essential essences are extracted. The oil is then placed over the water, and the water slowly cooked away, allowing the essences to mix with the oil (Yad, Kley HaMikdash 1:2; from Kerithoth 5a). According to another opinion, the oil was cooked with the aromatic herbs, and then filtered out."[8] I can't help but ponder on the former method of the herbs prepared by cooking in water and oil, because it sounds strikingly similar to a popular method I have personally used to prepare modern cannabis oil, with or without other herbs. This method is very effective for cleaning herbs of unwanted chlorophyll and fine plant debris in the final product.

Kanehbos[9] or kaneh bosem משב הנק also sounds like cannabis linguistically because the word *cannabis* is a linguistic derivative from the Hebrew, according to Rabbi Micheol Green in his article about the translation of the Hebrew, "Cannabis and the joys of biblical Hebrew!"[10]

Modern evidence for other uses of cannabis by ancient tribes of Judah can also be found in two very important discoveries. In 1993, an ancient skeleton of a girl who died in childbirth was found in a Jerusalem cave with a container of ashes bearing the chemical signature of cannabis phytocannabinoids. This container contained the ashes of cannabis that were burned for the girl, apparently used as a medicament during childbirth.[11] Then, in 2020, a

---

8   Kaplan, Aryeh. *The Living Torah,* http://bible.ort.org/books/pentd2.asp?ACTION=displaypage&BOOK =2&CHAPTER=30#C1800

9   "Cannabis," English to Hebrew translation, https://www.doitinhebrew.com/

10   Green, Micheol. "Cannabis and the joys of biblical Hebrew!" March 8, 2019, https://web.archive.org /web/20201119134549/https:/blogs.timesofisrael.com/cannabis-and-the-joys-of-biblical-hebrew/

11   Zias, J., H. Stark, J. Sellgman, R. Levy, E. Werker, A. Beuer, and R. Mechoulam. "Early medical use of cannabis." *Nature.* May 20, 1993. 363(6426):215. doi: 10.1038/363215a0. PMID: 8387642. https://www.nature .com/articles/363215a0.pdf

discovery of a Judahite shrine at Tel Arad contained evidence of incense offerings containing a dark residue with the chemical signatures of cannabis phytocannabinoids (specifically, THC, CBD, and CBN) and frankincense.[12]

In the Old Testament, we find that the holy anointing oil was strictly for the anointing of the priesthood and holy objects. But cannabis, as a stand-alone herb, was also used for medicine and as altar incense.

In the New Testament, Jesus and his disciples, who were also Jewish, carried forward the healing and worship practices that included cannabis by repurposing the holy anointing oil for personal devotion and to heal the sick.

King James Bible
Matthew 6:17 But thou, when thou fastest, anoint thine head, and wash thy face;
Mark 6:13 And they cast out many devils, and anointed with oil many that were sick, and healed them.
James 5:14 Is anyone among you sick? Let him call for the elders of the church, and let them pray over him, anointing him with oil in the name of the Lord.

In the last verse in this set of verses as read from the original Aramaic, the oil literally translates as "the meshkha," indicating a specific oil set apart for the purposes of anointing. In the other verses, *anoint* and *oil* are translated as "meshukh," the act of anointing the head (Matthew 6:17) and "meshkha" oil (Mark 6:13). Even more interesting, Jesus is called "Maran Eshu Meshikha," Our Lord Yeshua, the Anointed One. All are references to the specific oil and act of anointment with this oil.[13]

For the early Christians, gnostic Christians, this holy anointing oil (chrism) in the scripture plays the most important of roles:

---

12   Eran Arie, Baruch Rosen, and Dvory Namdar. *Cannabis and Frankincense at the Judahite Shrine of Arad,* Tel Aviv, 2020, 47:1, 5-28, DOI: 10.1080/03344355.2020.1732046 https://www.tandfonline.com/doi/full/10.1080/03344355.2020.1732046

13   Aramaic translation from https://www.thearamaicscriptures.com/

The Nag Hammadi
The Gospel of Philip
There is water within water and fire in the oil of chrism.

—

Through the Holy Spirit we are indeed begotten again, but we are begotten through Christ in the two. We are anointed through the Spirit. When we were begotten, we were united. None can see himself either in water or in a mirror without light. Nor again can you see in light without mirror or water. For this reason, it is fitting to baptize in the two, in the light and the water. Now the light is the chrism.

—

Philip the apostle said, "Joseph the carpenter planted a garden because he needed wood for his trade. It was he who made the cross from the trees which he planted. His own offspring hung on that which he planted. His offspring was Jesus, and the planting was the cross." But the Tree of Life is in the middle of the Garden. However, it is from the olive tree that we got the chrism, and from the chrism, the resurrection.

—

The chrism is superior to baptism, for it is from the word "Chrism" that we have been called "Christians," certainly not because of the word "baptism".
And it is because of the chrism that "the Christ" has his name. For the Father anointed the Son, and the Son anointed the apostles, and the apostles anointed us. He who has been anointed possesses everything. He possesses the resurrection, the light, the cross, the Holy Spirit. The Father gave him this in the bridal chamber; he merely accepted (the gift). The Father was in the Son and the Son in the Father. This is the Kingdom of Heaven.[14]

In India and China, we find historical evidence of the use of cannabis for mostly medicinal but also spiritual and euphoric purposes in many texts. Dr. William O'Shaughnessy, a

---

14   The Gospel of Philip, Translated by Wesley W. Isenberg, *The Nag Hammadi Library,* https://web.archive
.org/web/20211219013505/http://gnosis.org/naghamm/gop.html

world-renowned expert in the study of *Cannabis* ssp. *indica* in India and Indian culture, explains some of the many uses and his observations of the effects of cannabis in his own medical texts—but he is also a point of reference for many other authors of the period who wrote botanical and medical texts that included cannabis.

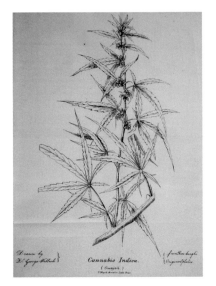

An illustration depicting the female *Cannabis* ssp. *indica* plant as seen in Dr. O'Shaughnessy's classic medical text from 1839, *On the preparations of the Indian hemp, or gunjah, (Cannabis Indica).*

"In the popular medicine of these nations, we find it extensively employed for a multitude of affections. But in western Europe its use either as a stimulant or as a remedy, is equally unknown. With the exception of the trial, as a frolic, of the Egyptian 'Hasheesh,' by a few youths in Marseilles, and of the clinical use of the wine of Hemp by Hahneman, as shewn in a subsequent extract, I have been unable to trace any notice of the employment of this drug in Europe."[15]

In Europe, the native cannabis species is a much taller and less resinous plant primarily used for fiber, namely rope and textiles, and oil seed production. This fact is noted by Dr. O'Shaughnessy and other botanical researchers of his era. In later chapters in the book *On the Preparations of the Indian Hemp, or Gunjah,* Dr. O'Shaughnessy does make note of some medicinal use of cannabis in Europe acquired from Egyptian sources.

In my own research, I have been unable to find any mention in these historical medical botany texts from the nineteenth century of a much earlier use of European *Cannabis* ssp. *sativa* as a medicament. The citation I was hoping to find actually comes from the research and writings of a German nun and physician, Hildegard of Bingen, in the twelfth century around 1151. Hildegard of Bingen's medical work was both experimental and visionary—and perhaps this spiritual quality of her medical texts would have been the reason it went unnoticed by the nineteenth- and early twentieth-century scientific community. Nonetheless, her prescription and advice for using the European hemp plant does not exclude

---

15 O'Shaughnessy, William. *On the Preparations of the Indian Hemp, or Gunjah,* (Cannabis Indica), *Their Effects on the Animal System in Health, and Their Utility in the Treatment of Tetanus and Other Convulsive Disorders.* 1839, 1.

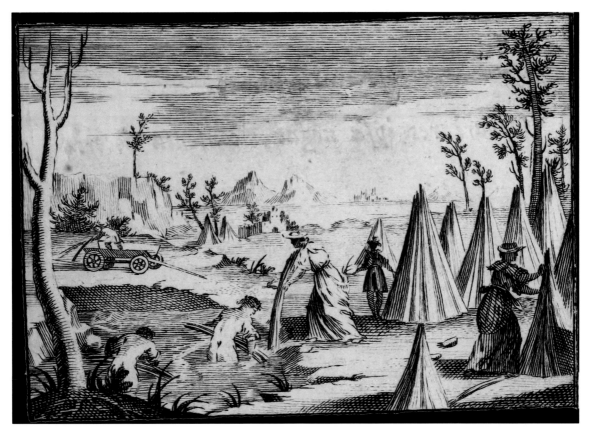

An illustration depicting hemp field production in the eighteenth century in Italy, from *Il Canapaio*, by Girolamo Baruffaldi, 1741.

European hemp as a psychoactive plant. Although this plant did not have the same hefty content of psychoactive phytocannabinoid (namely, THC), as *Cannabis* ssp. *indica,* she deemed it necessary to give a caveat for use with certain patients while extolling its medicinal value. And while topical use of *Cannabis* ssp. *indica* was known in the East, Bingen was the first to write about the topical use of cannabis hemp native to Europe.

"Hemp (hanff) is hot, and it grows where the air is neither very hot nor very cold, and its nature is similar. Its seed is salubrious, and good as food for healthy people. It is gentle and profitable to the stomach, taking away a bit of its mucus. It is easy to digest, diminishes bad humours, and fortifies good humours. Nevertheless, if one who is weak in the head, and has a vacant brain, eats hemp, it easily affects his head. It does not harm one who has a healthy head and full brain. If one is very ill, it even afflicts his stomach a bit. Eating it does not hurt one who is moderately ill.

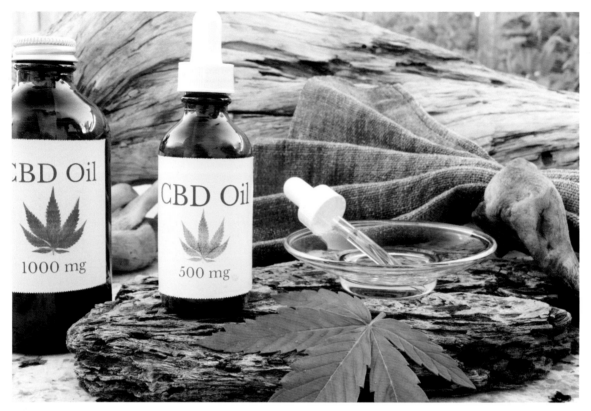

An example of a modern hemp fabric table napkin and hemp-derived CBD products for the mainstream retail market in the twenty-first century.

"Let one who has a cold stomach cook hemp in water and, when the water has been squeezed out, wrap it in a small cloth, and frequently place it warm, on his stomach. This strengthens and renews that area. Also a cloth made from hemp is good for binding ulcers and wounds, since the heat in it has been tempered."[16]

It's relevant to note that most of the cannabis hemp CBD derivative products so popular today primarily originate from the European *Cannabis* ssp. *sativa*. These would have been the cannabis plants Hildegard of Bingen worked with in her medical practices in Germany in the Middle Ages. While these European species of cannabis are low in euphoric compounds like THC, and higher in CBD, it would seem that Hildegard of Bingen recognized the potential for psychoactivity in the cannabis hemp native to Europe when she gave her caveat for use.

---

16 Von Bingen, Hildegard. *Physica*, 1158, 14, 1158, translation 1998 by Priscilla Throop.

We actually see this today in modern hemp farming. The federal government of the United States has legalized hemp for farming and commercial production since 2018, and defines *hemp* as any cannabis plant with no more than .30 percent THC content. Crops that turn "hot" (produce higher levels of THC) must be destroyed and are not allowed to come to market. It's not always predictable when the seeds are planted even with strains licensed for compliant THC levels. It's entirely possible to grow a hemp plant from European genetics that will produce enough THC to not only exceed the government hemp regulations, but also enough THC for a federally forbidden and mild euphoric experience.

Pre-Prohibition Material and Medicinal Use of Cannabis

Just imagine: if the US government had followed the advice of its own researchers and scientists, you would probably be reading this book printed on hemp paper right now! The US government effectively outlawed cannabis twenty-one years after this conclusion was published in this Department of Agriculture bulletin with the Marijuana Tax Act of 1937. Draw your own conclusions about the special interests that influenced this legislation in opposition to the most advanced scientific and medical research available at that time.

For centuries up until prohibition, hemp had been used to make the highest-quality and most durable products—not just paper, but also rope, fabric, insulation, sails for ships, building materials, fuel oils, and more! Our ancestors used hemp in everyday

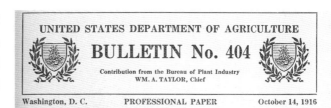

Cover for an official US Government Department of Agriculture bulletin from 1916 detailing research conducted into hemp paper making.

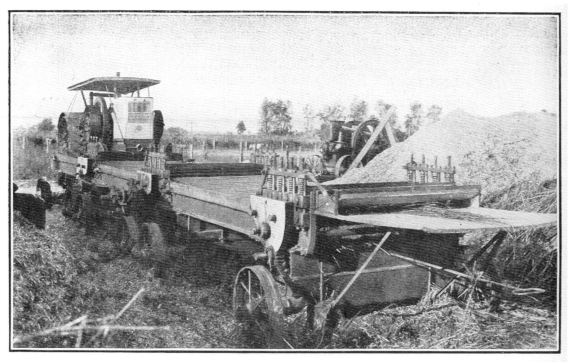

FIG. 2.—Machine brake and hemp hurds. Hemp hurds from machine brakes quickly accumulate in large piles.

A photograph of hemp field machine production of hemp hurds for papermaking from the same 1916 bulletin.

CONCLUSIONS.

There appears to be little doubt that under the present system of forest use and consumption the present supply can not withstand the demands placed upon it. By the time improved methods of forestry have established an equilibrium between production and consumption, the price of pulp wood may be such that a knowledge of other available raw materials may be imperative.

Semicommercial paper-making tests were conducted, therefore, on hemp hurds, in cooperation with a paper manufacturer. After several trials, under conditions of treatment and manufacture which are regarded as favorable in comparison with those used with pulp wood, paper was produced which received very favorable comment both from investigators and from the trade and which according to official tests would be classed as a No. 1 machine-finish printing paper.

The official conclusion of the research studies detailed in the 1916 bulletin: hemp makes the best quality paper and most sustainable paper and is far superior to wood pulp paper.

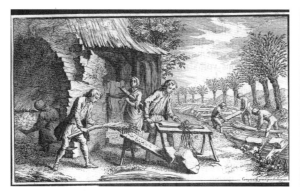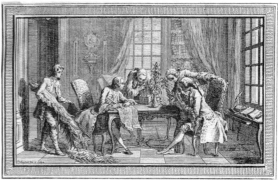

From *Traité de la fabrique des manœuvres pour les vaisseaux, ou, L'art de la corderie perfectionné*, by Duhamel du Monceau, M., Soubeyran, Pierre, Basseporte, Madeleine-Françoise, 1747. These illustrations depict fresh hemp farmers harvesting and processing their crop, and hemp merchants examining hemp plants and harvested plant samples for fiber qualities.

life for material use, food, and medicine. Hemp as an expensive or "specialty" item is an artifact of prohibition in the modern world and not a true representation of the actual costs to produce and process it. But someday, hemp could very well once again become a sustainable part of our daily lives.

Our pharmaceutical companies knew what the ancients knew about the effectiveness and benefits of using cannabis for many ailments and symptom management. Cannabis was a reliable and effective medicine that had been in use for thousands of years before the pharmaceutical companies applied their labels to extracts and blends of cannabis with other ingredients.

Most medical reference volumes published for use by doctors in the nineteenth and early twentieth century included cannabis as a treatment for a variety of conditions, with analgesia being one of the most common uses. In the 1922 medical reference encyclopedias for physicians *Analytic Cyclopedia of Practical Medicine* by Charles Sajous, MD, the exceptional benefits of cannabis as an analgesic are noted for a number of painful conditions, including spasmodic dysmenorrhea (menstrual cramping), and touted as a safer alternative to morphine. Dr. Sajous cites and notes the following:

> Cannabis indica has come into widespread use as a remedy for pain of various kinds, more especially in the headaches attending migraine, eye-strain, the menopause, and even brain tumors or uremia.

No. 183. INDIAN-HEMP, FOREIGN, U. S. P., 1880
(Assayed).

(CANNABIS INDICA.)

The dried Flowering Top of Cannabis Sativa.

(Contains not less than 10 per cent. of dry extractive matter.)

NATURAL ORDER.—Urticaceæ, Cannabineæ.
HABITAT.—Asia, India.
COMMON NAMES.—Cannabis Indica, Hashish, Churrus Gunja.
ACTIVE CONSTITUENTS.—Resin, Choline or Neurine.

Medicinally, this drug is a powerful narcotic, producing, when first given, exhilaration and intoxication, and subsequently, drowsiness and stupor. It is said to act as a decided aphrodisiac, and is preferable to opium in causing sleep, allaying spasms and relieving pain, without the usual disturbing after-effects of the latter, such as nauseating the stomach or constipating the bowels.

Antidotes.—In case of an over-dose, hot brandy and water may be given, vegetable acids, such as lemon juice or vinegar, and the patient be allowed to sleep. A blister to the nape of the neck is recommended to control its violent action.

Dose.—2 to 5 minims (0.12—0.30 c. c.), on a lump of sugar.

PREPARATIONS.

Tincture of Foreign Indian-Hemp, U. S. P., 1880.

Fluid Extract	2¾ fluid ounces (82.50 c. c.)
Alcohol	13¼ fluid ounces (397.50 c. c.)

M. and filter. *Dose.*—20 to 30 minims (1.25—1.90 c. c.).

Infusion of Foreign Indian-Hemp.

Fluid Extract	½ fluid ounce (15. c. c.)
Hot Water	16 fluid ounces (480. c. c.)

M. Useful as a lotion to painful tumors.

From the 1892 pharmaceutical catalog of John Wyeth & Brother, also known as Wyeth Pharmaceuticals, and in 2009 acquired by Pfizer Inc., manufactured a full-spectrum, whole plant, cannabis medicine for both internal and external use, like many other pharmaceutical companies of the era, until this medication was discontinued after legislative measures were enacted to prohibit cannabis in all forms, including as a medicine, in the twentieth century.

FL. EXT. CANNABIS INDICA........................Dose 5 to 60 m.

Cannabis sativa Linn. var. *indica,*   **Nat. Ord.**—*Urticaceæ.*

Synonyms—Cannabis sativa Linn.,—Indian cannabis, U. S.,—Foreign indian hemp, Gunjah, Hashish, Churrus, Bhang, Subjer.

Range—Caucasus, Persia, Northern India; cultivated in Europe, Asia and the United States.

Habitat—Rich moist soil of mountain slopes and banks of streams.

Part used—The inflorescence of the female plant.

Standard of strength—5 c.c. evaporated to dryness at 212° F., yields a residue weighing 0.65 grams.

Action and uses—NOT POISONOUS according to best authorities, though formerly so regarded. Antispasmodic, analgesic, anesthetic, narcotic, aphrodisiac. Specially recommended in spasmodic and painful affections; for preventing rather than arresting migraine; almost a specific in that form of insanity peculiar to women, caused by mental worry or moral shock. It is the best hypnotic in delirium tremens. Its anodyne power is marked in chronic metritis and dysmenorrhea. Used with excellent results in habitues of opium, chloral or cocaine. In hysterical cases not calmed by chloral or opium it acts especially well,

PREPARATION.

Tincture Cannabis Indica, U. S.—Fl. ext. Cannabis indica, Lilly, 2⅜ fl. ozs.; Alcohol, 13⅝ fl. ozs.; Mix—Dose 30 minims increased till its effects are experienced.

From the 1897 Eli Lilly pharmaceutical handbook, one of a dozen cannabis medicines and medicine blends manufactured by Eli Lilly in the late nineteenth century. Almost every pharmaceutical company of the period had their own cannabis formulary, and all of these medicines were included in the official U.S.P. as legitimate medicines of the period.

LIEBIG'S CORN CURE.

The following formula for Liebig's Corn Cure is said to be very effective:

Take of—

> Extract of cannabis indica ... 5 parts.
> Salicylic acid............... 30 parts.
> Collodion ....240 parts.

Mix until dissolved. Apply with a camel-hair pencil four consecutive nights and mornings to form a thick coating. The collodion protects the corn from irritation and rubbing, while the extract of cannabis indica acts as an anodyne, and the salicylic acid dissolves and disintegrates the corn.

From *Secret nostrums and systems of medicine, A Book of Formulas,* by Charles W. Oleson, MD, 1890. This book was a formulary for compounding pharmacies and doctors. The corn treatment detailed in this recipe was a commercial medicine sold over the counter at the time, but a pharmacist could also compound it from this recipe if needed. Cannabis was used as a topical treatment for the relief of pain while the other ingredient, salicylic acid, dissolved the corn and the colloidal ingredient protected the skin.

Moderate use produces no injurious effects on the mind, except in cases of marked neurotic diathesis. Excessive use both indicates and intensifies mental instability. It tends to weaken the mind, and may even lead to insanity, especially in cases where there is already weakness or hereditary predisposition. Report of Indian Hemp Drugs Commission (*Therap.Gaz.*, April 1905). There is no proof that cannabis indica extract by itself, taken internally or even smoked, causes a habit, and to continue to list it with such habit forming drugs as morphine, chloral, and alcohol greatly detracts from whatever value it might possess as a sedative. M. V. Ball (*Therap. Gaz.*, Nov., 1910)."[17]

But the work of botanical researchers, doctors, and scientists of the nineteenth century and earlier who wrote so much about cannabis came to a close when prohibition became a focus in the early twentieth century as a viable and progressive solution for what was viewed as the moral degradation of society. Perhaps we can speculate with some accuracy, based on the evidence presented in this chapter, that the authentic rationale for prohibition was likely to ensure that other competing interests, such as logging and more profitable pharmaceuticals, had a better seat at the economic table. Medical cannabis research would not be picked up again until the 1960s in Israel when Dr. Raphael Mechoulam began his groundbreaking work in cannabis phytocannabinoid research.

Cannabis was not grown again in the United States in the twentieth century except for a small fraction of the previous crop production during the Second World War for rope and other necessary fiber needed for the war effort. After the war, all cannabis farming was officially discontinued until hemp was re-legalized again by the federal government with The Hemp Farming Act of 2018. As of 2022, thirty-eight individual states, six tribal nations, and four territories have legalized whole-plant cannabis in some form, including the psychoactive varieties of cannabis, for both medicinal and commercial retail markets.[18]

---

17 Sajous, Charles. *Sajous Analytic Cyclopedia of Practical Medicine Volume 3,* 1922, 6–7.
18 "Legality of Cannabis by U.S. jurisdiction." Wikipedia. https://en.wikipedia.org/wiki/Legality_of_cannabis _by_U.S._jurisdiction

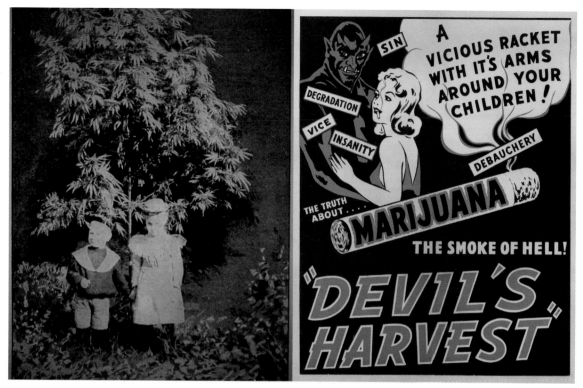

From left to right: Children holding hands in front of a cannabis plant as seen in the book hemp (*Cannabis sativa*) by Sindey Smith Boyce, publication date 1900. Circa year 1942, a movie poster for *Devil's Harvest* by Director Ray Test and Writer Edward Clark, one of many cannabis exploitation and scaremongering propaganda films and books produced in the early decades of the twentieth century to ensure public acceptance of the prohibition of cannabis in the United States, after several legislative measures, including the Marihuana Tax Act of 1937.

The Absurdity of "Illegal" Plants Rediscovered in the Twenty-First Century

In the early twentieth century, after centuries of use as a fiber crop, food crop, and for both medicine and spiritual ecstasy in many places around the globe, including North America, this legitimate, family-friendly crop and medicinal plant preparation found in every pharmacy in the United States became vilified as a "drug" used by "Mexicans" and "jazz musicians," and condemned as a "gateway" leading to destruction.

The unfortunate legacy of the "gateway" mythology persists to this day in law enforcement, the prison system, the clergy, education, and in public health policy—but this is changing! A more balanced viewpoint about cannabis that existed more than one hundred years ago is once again coming back into focus in the twenty-first century with the repeal of cannabis prohibition in many locations. Prohibition of other plants and fungi once considered moral scourges and criminal vices is also being repealed as the expensive and failed "Drug War" of the twentieth century comes to a close.

The concept of "illegal" plants is, and always has been, an absurd concept—with the closest approximation to the twentieth-century "Drug War" taking place during the latter Middle Ages when thousands of people, mostly women, were persecuted, tortured, and murdered for practicing "witchcraft." Many of these innocent people were women who were adept community herbalists practicing at a time when ignorance flourished and life was often brutal and short due to lack of scientific knowledge. It was a dangerous time to be an old woman outside the institution of the church who was knowledgeable about the medicinal properties of herbs and foods.[19]

I've often wondered why it is that some plants are illegal and some plants are legal. And how ironic it was that, right next door

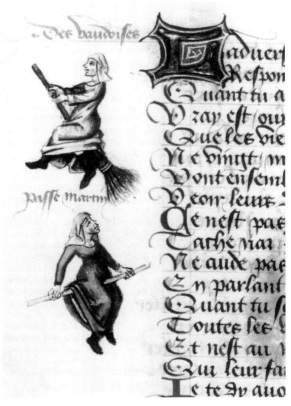

Martin Le Franc's "Ladies' Champion," 1451. Of great concern to the church authorities in the Middle Ages were the flying ointments of "witches." These ointments contained ingredients still in use today in modern chemistry but that had the reputation during the Middle Ages of enabling witches to fly. Some of the combinations of ingredients in these ointments may have had hallucinogenic properties. No doubt, a free woman making ointments for the purposes of healing flights was a grave offense in the eyes of the male clergy.[20]

to the elementary school in a town I lived in several years ago, there was a field with poison

19 Minkowski, W. L. "Women healers of the middle ages: selected aspects of their history." *American Journal of Public Health*, 82(2), 1992, 288–295. https://doi.org/10.2105/ajph.82.2.288

20 Thompsom, Helen. "How Witches' Brews Helped Bring Modern Drugs to Market." *Smithsonian Magazine*, 2014. https://www.smithsonianmag.com/science-nature/how-witches-brews-helped-bring-modern-drugs-market-180953202/

hemlock (*Conium maculatum*) that flourished untouched. Law enforcement or school administrators didn't seem to mind that a field of plants capable of killing a curious child, or two, or three who may consume a very small portion of the flowers or leaves was ever present. I'm fairly certain that none of them knew what this flowering herb was growing next to the playground. Poison hemlock escapes the watchful eyes of the watchers because it isn't "euphoric" when consumed, and therefore not "illegal" or "dangerous for children." The legal status of any given plant would appear to have nothing at all to do with how lethal it is for humans or animals. Perhaps the solution is that we should be teaching more botany lessons in school and at home and stop waging war on plants.

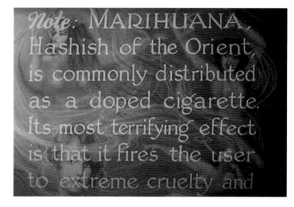

A still from the 1936 propaganda film *Marihuana*. The prohibitionist mythology about the cannabis plant hasn't changed at all in eighty-seven years. The key difference in modern professional prohibitionism is that prohibitionists are careful to excise the racist terminology and beef up the alarmism with their own "researchers and clinicians" who carry the same biases as yesteryear papered over with scientific or medical "authority" instead of naked nymphs frolicking in the smoke of the devil's lettuce.

It's interesting to consider that the more prohibitionist propaganda has progressed with the times, the more it operates the same as it always has, promoting the same message it always does, even in 2023.

In the twenty-first century, professional prohibitionists have publicized many successful alarmist propaganda campaigns, but the one that always seems to stir the most dysphoria in the anxious public is the repetition of the "cannabis is stronger nowadays" and "this isn't the cannabis your grandfather smoked at Woodstock" myth.

This is perhaps the most easily debunked myth that is promoted, so much so that it's baffling when I see it go unchallenged.

Depending on who your grandfather knew at Woodstock, he could have been smoking the infamous Acapulco Red, Thai Stick, or Colombian Gold—legendary strains of cannabis from the sixties and seventies that rival many of the strains found in legal cannabis dispensaries of today. Your grandfather could have been smoking Moroccan hashish, too, a concentrated cannabis resin product with a soaring THC content of 40 percent or more.

Many of the new strains of cannabis available today descended from the phytocan-nabinoid-rich landraces of yesteryear. The cannabis plant cannot produce more than 30 percent of its weight in resins. Most top-shelf strains of cannabis found in today's modern dispensaries tops out at 25 percent THC. And 20 percent is much more common than 25 percent. But most mid-shelf retail cannabis flowers are going to be somewhere in the range of 15 percent to 18 percent THC. If your grandfather smoked Thai Stick at Woodstock, or even Thai Stick of the 1980s (I smoked Thai Stick in the 1980s), what he was smoking was as potent as most of the cannabis offered in a modern, legal dispensary.

Cannabis isn't "stronger" today. Cannabis strains previously unavailable for mass distribution, and cannabis strains developed from those legendary landrace strains, are more available than ever.

And there are more opportunities in legal cannabis dispensaries and legal home growing than ever to market and grow cannabis completely free of euphoric effects like CBD and CBG-rich cannabis strains. There is a prodigious customer base clamoring for "the cannabis that doesn't get you high"—this was unheard of in the prohibition era. That's the real difference between today's cannabis and "the cannabis at Woodstock." Nonpsychoactive cannabis products and plant strains are the most popular cannabis products of all in the twenty-first century.

It's true that modern cannabis dispensaries do not sell the low-potency, crusty, brick "dirt weed" that was also available on the black market during the prohibition years. And that's actually a good thing, because cannabis of questionable quality and phytocannabinoid potency poses risks to human health, such as drug, mold, and pesticide contamination. Cannabis that is found in the legal modern dispensaries of today has passed through several testing hoops that include not only phytocannabinoid content measurement, but testing for mold, pesticides, adulteration, and heavy metals, too. Cannabis isn't "stronger" today; cannabis is safer today.

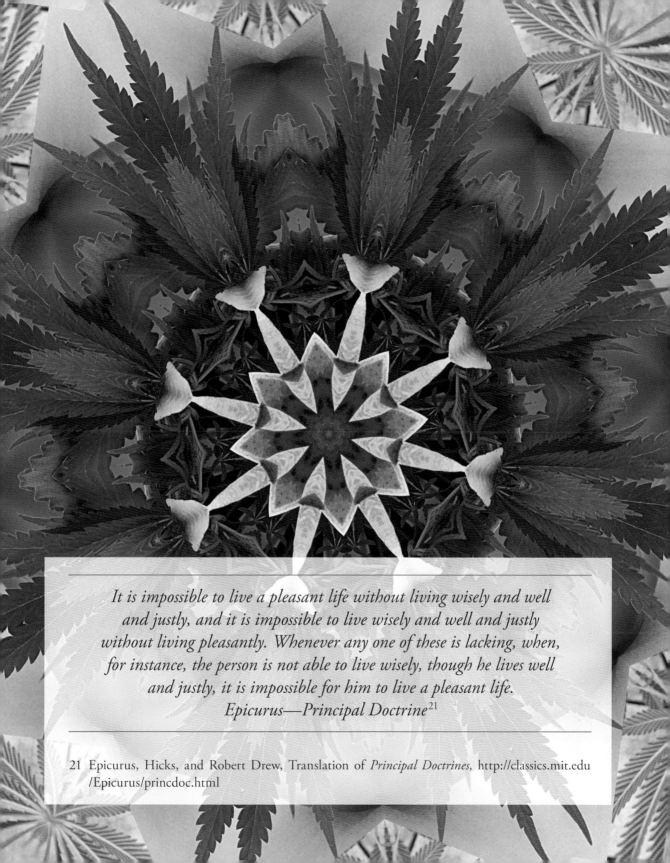

It is impossible to live a pleasant life without living wisely and well
and justly, and it is impossible to live wisely and well and justly
without living pleasantly. Whenever any one of these is lacking, when,
for instance, the person is not able to live wisely, though he lives well
and justly, it is impossible for him to live a pleasant life.
Epicurus—Principal Doctrine[21]

21 Epicurus, Hicks, and Robert Drew, Translation of *Principal Doctrines,* http://classics.mit.edu
/Epicurus/princdoc.html

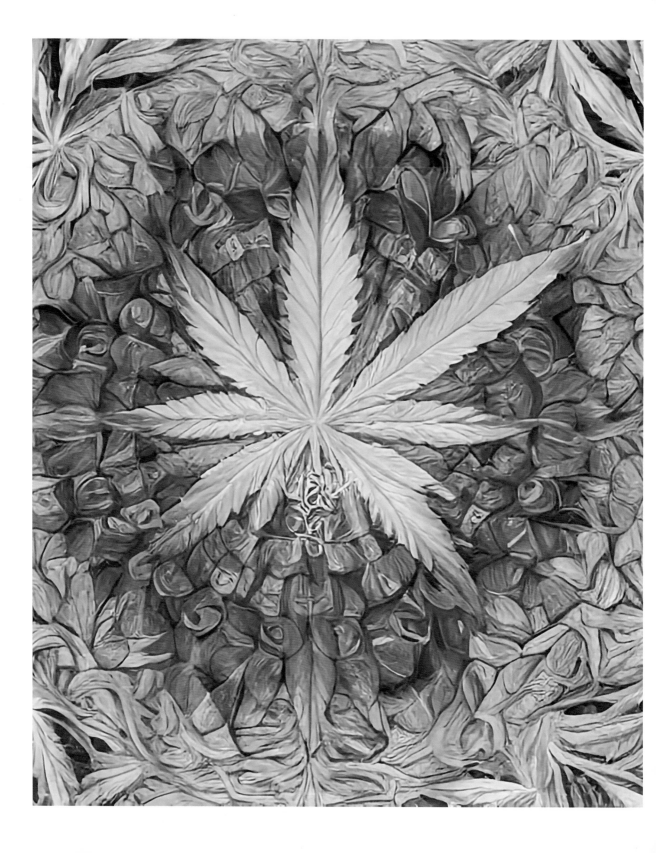

CHAPTER TWO

TREK INTO THE WEEDS: THE BASICS OF CANNABIS CHEMISTRY AND BOTANY

In this chapter, we will have a simple overview of the chemistry of cannabis plants, the botany of male, female, and hermaphrodite cannabis plants, and finally, you'll learn a simple step-by-step method for growing your first cannabis plant. Now that cannabis has been legalized for both medicine and pleasure in many locations, it's possible to grow this once-contraband crop at home. If home growing is legal where you live, then growing one female plant is a fun way to learn basic hands-on cannabis botany.

Cannabis Anatomy and Plant Identification

Cannabis sativa L., and all its subspecies, such as *Cannabis* ssp. *indica,* and all hybrids, are dioecious plants, as male and female flowers are typically produced on different plants. Throughout history, cannabis has been interchangeably called hemp, Indian hemp, cannabis, and marijuana. These are all the same species, the same plant, if you will, which has thousands of hybrids due mostly to human intervention—but some of these also occur naturally in the wild.

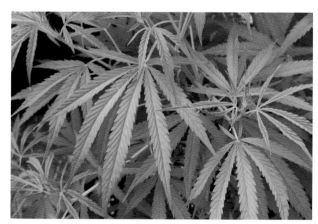

The vegetation stage of a cannabis plant. All cannabis plants look like this until the seasonal photoperiod changes to late summer and fall, unless the plant is from the *Cannabis* ssp. *ruderalis* species, which will go to flower based on developmental age instead of photoperiod. If grown indoors, the cannabis plant will look like this until the artificial lighting is adjusted to reflect a shorter day, which is typically twelve hours of light. The vegetation stage typically requires sixteen to eighteen hours of light. The leaves in the veg stage are also known as "fan leaves" and contain very few, if any, trichomes.

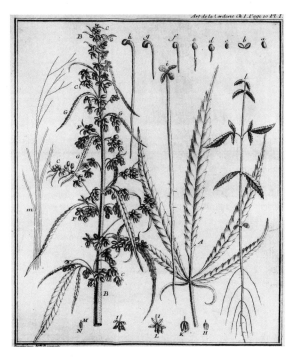
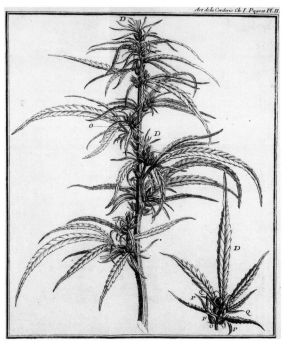

Cannabis sativa L. Illustration of male and female cannabis anatomy from *Traité de la fabrique des manœuvres pour les vaisseaux, ou, L'art de la corderie perfectionné,* by Duhamel du Monceau, M., Soubeyran, Pierre, Basseporte, Madeleine-Françoise, 1747. A text in the fine art of rope production from France. Cannabis was long favored as a superior fiber from which to manufacture rope for utilitarian and decorative use.

Illustration Key

Left: A male cannabis plant with anatomy and growing stages from seed to seedling.

A—A cannabis fan leaf

B, B—The main top stem of the male cannabis plant showing the abundance of male flowers

C, F, G—The male flowers as they grow in bunches from the stem nodes

H—A closed male flower bud

K—A male flower bud almost ready to open

I—A fully opened male flower bud

L—Stamens of the fully opened male flower bud

M, N—Single male flower petal with stamen

a—A single seed

b—The seed coat

c—Interior of the seed, including root cap, cotyledons, radicle, primary leaves, shoot apex

d, e, f, g, h—Emergence of seedling stages starting with radicle, and cotyledons

i—The seedling showing the cotyledon leaves and the emergence of the primary leaves of the plant and the lateral roots that begin to develop.

l—A cannabis plant that has moved from the seedling stage to the vegetation stage.

m—The interior of the stem showing the fibers

Right: A flowering female cannabis plant

D—Main top stem of the flowering female cannabis plant

F—Seed calyx and stigma formation with bracts

O—Female flower stem as it emerges from a main stem node

P, Q—Sugar leaves and bracts emerging from female cannabis flowers

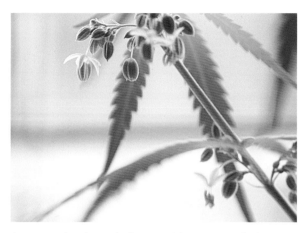

An example of a male flower with many small clusters of buds ready to open and release pollen. Male cannabis flowers look strikingly different from female cannabis flowers and typically have sparser growth than the compact and lush female flower.

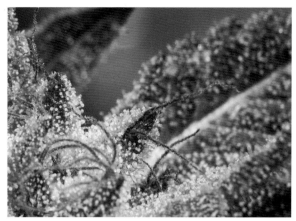

This is a close-up of the cannabis trichomes. The trichome is the hairlike gland producing all of the phytocannabinoids, terpenes, and a few other cannabis compounds. The trichomes are resinous and feel sticky when touched.

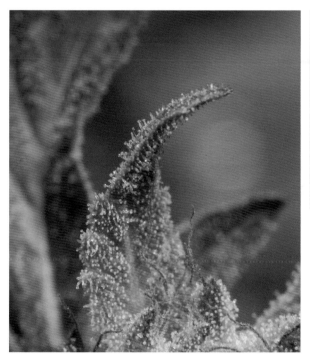

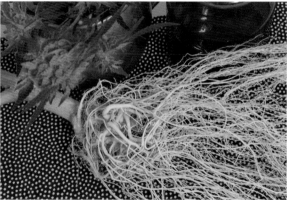

Like most other seed-bearing plants, cannabis has an underground root system that nourishes the aboveground parts of the plant. This root system has many uses, both as a culinary enhancer in savory foods and a popular ingredient in some medicinal salve and tincture products. It does not contain psychoactive properties.

Sugar leaves form as part of the flower bracts that develop as the cannabis flower matures and fills out. These leaves, being part of the flower, are also rich in trichomes, unlike the fan leaves.

Females, Males, Hermaphrodites, and Simple Genetics

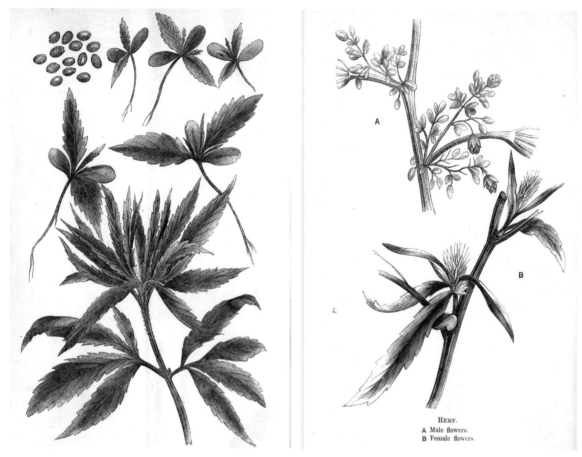

HEMP.
A Male flowers.
B Female flowers.

From *Flax and hemp, their culture and manipulation*, by E. Sebastian Delamer, 1854, an instructional manual on growing and processing both flax and hemp. These illustrations represent two stages of cannabis growth, (left) the vegetation stage and (right) the flowering stage of both males and females.

Each cannabis seed, unless feminized, will produce either a male or female plant. Male plants have the lowest amount of resinous phytocannabinoid, and females, especially when bred alone and away from males, have the highest amount of resinous phytocannabinoid. You will not be able to predict from the size or shape of a seed, or any other characteristic of the seed, whether the plant is destined to become male or female.

Apart from pollen production for the purposes of making fresh seeds for breeding programs, male cannabis plants will probably have limited use for a beginner. The roots can be used to make various preparations calling for cannabis roots, and the leaves can be used as a nonintoxicating green vegetable. Some of these uses are described in chapter 6, on using cannabis as a nonpsychoactive green vegetable.

But wait! There's actually one more kind of cannabis plant: the hermaphrodite. These cannabis plants, due to a variety of reasons, have a genetic or environmental cause behind their production of both male and female flowers on the same plant.

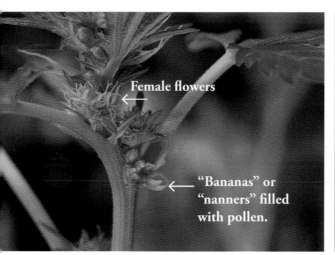
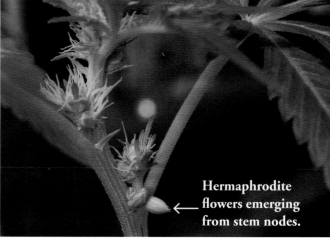

A cannabis plant displaying both male and female flowers like this one is called a hermaphrodite or "hermie."

This hermaphrodite plant will seed itself and produce female seed. However, this seed is not a good seed for growing female cannabis plants, as the plants will have weaknesses, and they are very likely to also become hermaphrodites. There is only one exception to this rule: if hermaphroditism is chemically induced using colloidal silver to produce only feminized seeds, then the genetics should be stable and not produce many, if any at all, hermaphrodite offspring.

Cannabis Chemistry Basics

What happens inside a cannabis plant? Let's have a look:

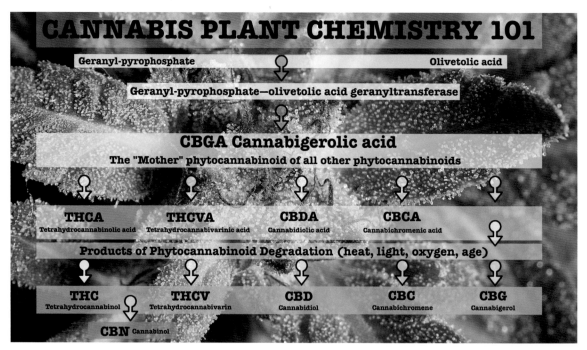

CANNABIS PLANT CHEMISTRY 101

Geranyl-pyrophosphate → Olivetolic acid

Geranyl-pyrophosphate—olivetolic acid geranyltransferase

CBGA Cannabigerolic acid
The "Mother" phytocannabinoid of all other phytocannabinoids

THCA	THCVA	CBDA	CBCA
Tetrahydrocannabinolic acid	Tetrahydrocannabivarinic acid	Cannabidiolic acid	Cannabichromenic acid

Products of Phytocannabinoid Degradation (heat, light, oxygen, age)

THC	THCV	CBD	CBC	CBG
Tetrahydrocannabinol	Tetrahydrocannabivarin	Cannabidiol	Cannabichromene	Cannabigerol

CBN Cannabinol

A simple flowchart showing the basic pathway in cannabis for making phytocannabinoids.[1] Cannabis actually makes more than one hundred phytocannabinoids, and when you count all the terpenes and other compounds produced by the plant, the total of all compounds is more than four hundred. Most of these compounds occur in trace amounts. Many of these compounds are still not well understood. Thanks to the changing legal status of cannabis, research continues in the area of identification and purposes that these compounds serve for the cannabis plant and how they can be used to benefit humans and animals.[2]

1   Wróbel, Thomasz, Mariola Dreger, Karoline Wielgus, and Ryszard Slmoski. "The application of plant in vitro cultures in cannabinoid production." *Biotechnology Letters.* 2018, 40. 10.1007/s10529-017 -2492-1. https://www.researchgate.net/publication/321860070_The_application_of_plant_in_vitro_cultures _in_cannabinoid_production

2   Oier Aizpurua-Olaizola, Umut Soydaner, Ekin Öztürk, Daniele Schibano, Yilmaz Simsir, Patricia Navarro, Nestor Etxebarria, and Aresatz Usobiaga, "Evolution of the Cannabinoid and Terpene Content during the Growth of Cannabis sativa Plants from Different Chemotypes." *Journal of Natural Products.* 2016. 79 (2), 324–331 DOI: 10.1021/acs.jnatprod.5b00949 https://pubs.acs.org/doi/abs/10.1021/acs .jnatprod.5b00949

In this brief overview of cannabis chemistry, we are going to explore the eleven most common phytocannabinoids that will be encountered when growing your own cannabis or when purchasing cannabis at a dispensary. These are the phytocannabinoids that occur in the largest amounts and make up the majority of phytocannabinoid content of the cannabis plant. The phytocannabinoid profile of any individual cannabis plant depends on a few factors, genetics, growth, harvest, processing, and aging.

Many people who are cannabis greenhorns are surprised to learn that cannabis doesn't produce many of their favorite phytocannabinoids directly! CBD is one example of this. CBD is not actually made by the cannabis plant; it occurs as a process of degradation of the CBDA molecule produced by the cannabis plant. The way this happens with CBD, and other degraded phytocannabinoids like THC, THCV, CBG, and CBC, is that the phytocannabinoid produced by the cannabis plant loses carbon atoms in a process known as decarboxylation. This changes the CBDA from cannabidiolic acid into CBD cannabidiol. This process happens through exposure to heat, light, oxygen, and age. The acidic phytocannabinoids produced by cannabis are delicate and lose carbon atoms quite readily via exposure.

Decarboxylation is when the natural acidic phytocannabinoids like THCA, CBDA, and CBGA produced naturally by the cannabis plant lose carbon atoms via the process of degradation (exposure to heat, light, oxygen, and aging, or a combination of these exposures) to become the phytocannabinoids that we are most familiar with, like THC, CBD, and CBG. **The cannabis plant does not directly produce any of the euphoric phytocannabinoids directly! These phytocannabinoids (THC, THCV, CBN) are produced only after decarboxylation of the directly produced acidic precursors of THCA and THCVA.**

Let's take a look at each of the five major phytocannabinoids produced in cannabis, their six phytocannabinoid products of decarboxylation/degradation, their availability, and some of their effects:

Regarding the legality of various phytocannabinoids, this is dependent upon the laws and regulations of the specific locale you are in. In 2018, hemp farming and hemp production was legalized under federal law in the United States. Even though hemp and the more euphoric varieties of cannabis are the same plant, the US government defines hemp as any *Cannabis sativa* L. plant measuring less than 0.30 percent THC. Any product produced from a cannabis plant with less than 0.30 percent THC is legal under federal law at this time as of 2022.

Specific laws vary from state to state, and country to country, and while cannabis plants considered "hemp" may be legal under US federal law, states may have different laws and regulations regarding this matter. Always check on the specific laws of your locale to determine the legality of purchase, possession, and use of cannabinoids or growing cannabis.

CBGA / Cannabigerolic acid: This is the mother phytocannabinoid of all other phytocannabinoids that occur in the cannabis plant. The cannabis plant produces this phytocannabinoid first, and over time, as the plant matures, CBGA transforms into all of the other phytocannabinoids. Most cannabis plants have very low levels of CBGA at harvesttime. To increase CBGA/CBG levels, cannabis plants are typically harvested early. This will mean that the other phytocannabinoids will not be as prolific. A few hemp strains have recently been developed in favor of CBGA/CBG production specifically.

It is purported to have many of the same benefits as THC, but without any euphoric, potentially psychedelic, or potentially intoxicating effects. CBGA is used as pain relief and inflammation relief similar to CBDA. Antiviral activity has also been reported.[3] Like other phytocannabinoids produced directly by the cannabis plant, this is an unstable molecule and easily converts to CBG with exposure. Capturing this molecule requires careful extraction and storage away from exposure to heat, light, and oxygen. CBGA is best captured from fresh cannabis flowers, carefully extracted, carefully stored, and used quickly (within three months). As of 2022, CBGA is federally legal in the United States if it is derived from hemp.

CBG / Cannabigerol: This phytocannabinoid is a direct degradation product of CBGA. CBG occurs when CBGA does not go on to develop into the other phytocannabinoids but is harvested and subject to exposure, usually heat, to transform it into CBG. CBGA and CBG have similar activity profiles and are not euphoric, potentially psychedelic, or potentially intoxicating; however, many anecdotes about CBG have described a very mild effect similar

---

3   Oregon State Research Shows Hemp Compounds Prevent Coronavirus from Entering Human Cells," Jan. 2022, Steve Lundeberg, https://today.oregonstate.edu/news/oregon-state-research-shows-hemp-compounds-prevent-coronavirus-entering-human-cells

to coffee in terms of psychoactivity. As of 2022, CBG is federally legal in the United States if it is derived from hemp.

CBDA / Cannabidiolic acid: This is the precursor molecule produced directly by the cannabis plant for the decarboxylated phytocannabinoid, CBD. It has many of the same properties attributed to CBD, but it appears to be more effective for applications such as pain relief when paired with CBD and other entourage compounds.[4] Capturing this molecule requires careful extraction and careful storage away from exposure to heat, light, and oxygen. CBDA is best captured from fresh cannabis flowers, carefully extracted, carefully stored, and used quickly (within three months). CBDA is not euphoric, potentially psychedelic, or potentially intoxicating. As of 2022, CBDA is federally legal in the United States if it is derived from hemp.

CBD / Cannabidiol: This phytocannabinoid product has been ubiquitous in the retail market for the past few years and remains so as of 2022. CBD is a unique phytocannabinoid in the United States in that it is both a FDA-approved prescription medicine for seizures, under the trade name of Epidiolex,[5] and a federally legal derivative of hemp sold on the consumer-level retail market as personal care and beauty products. People who use CBD as an herbal preparation do so for a variety of reasons. Some of these reasons are based on legitimate scientific evidence, and some are based on dubious claims made by product manufacturers.

CBD is also a common phytocannabinoid that can be purchased in state-legal medical and adult-use cannabis dispensaries. The CBD sold in state-legal dispensaries is typically full-spectrum and derived from the whole flowers and trim of state-legal cannabis plants. Unlike the mainstream retail market, the plants do not have to meet the federal maximum limits of 0.30 percent THC, and these products are strictly regulated by the state. Many CBD products found in state-legal cannabis dispensaries may also be combined with THC and other phytocannabinoids.

Most federally legal, hemp-derived CBD sold at the retail level is known as CBD isolate, which is readily purchased in wholesale bulk quantities at often rock-bottom prices. CBD isolate is the singular CBD molecule that has been chemically stripped from

---

4   Kogan, Mikhail, MD, and Joan Liebmann-Smith. "Cannabis Treatment for Aches and Pains." ProjectCBD. https://www.projectcbd.org/cannabis-treatment-aches-pains

5   Epidiolex Official Website. https://www.epidiolex.com/

hemp resin. It's often added to cheap bulk bases such as tinctures, oils, lotions, and edibles, and sold for astronomical prices in mainstream retail stores in almost every state in the United States and many other countries. CBD is sold in isolated form in the retail market in order to serve consumers who want or need a product totally free of THC, which is even more stringent than the federally legal maximum THC content of 0.30 percent. This is an enormous consumer base—much larger than the consumer base for whole-spectrum or raw flower CBD from state-legal cannabis dispensaries and the number of people who grow their own CBD cannabis strains.

There is a lot of debate about the effectiveness of this stripped-down cannabinoid devoid of its naturally occurring entourage compounds. Many of these retail products are made with artificial ingredients like synthetic fragrances. Many of the manufacturers don't even attempt to formulate an "entourage" structure around the isolated CBD molecule. And as we know from numerous studies, it is the entourage effect that increases the effectiveness of phytocannabinoids.[6] "Hemp" or "CBD" is slapped on a label as the predominant selling point for the product, and the quality of the formulation and ingredients takes a back seat to modern CBD hype. Many of these products also target senior citizens and the chronically ill who live in states without access to state-regulated legal cannabis products and dispensaries. Many of these products that have been shown to contain little to no CBD as well as being adulterated with toxins such as lead and mold.[7]

More than any other cannabis-derived product, CBD isolate products are often at the center of many fraudulent claims and products.

When you put the pricing of wholesale bulk CBD isolate into perspective with the cost of the base ingredients, even high-quality base ingredients, an eighty-dollar price tag for a one-ounce jar of salve or bottle of oil just doesn't make sense for this kind of product in most cases—and, unfortunately, this is the level of pricing for many of these CBD-isolate products.

Another caveat when purchasing CBD products is to be wary of any CBD product that claims to be produced from any other plants. Unfalsifiable claims about plants that make CBD which are not cannabis are made in order to avoid the ongoing stigma regarding

---

6   Kogan, MD, Mikhail and Joan Liebmann-Smith PhD. "Cannabis Treatment for Aches and Pains." ProjectCBD. https://www.projectcbd.org/cannabis-treatment-aches-pains.

7   "Stop CBD Scams From Stealing Your Money With Dr. Phil" https://www.youtube.com/watch?v=a4ZXs94e018 Feb. 17 2021

cannabis in some locations. Makers and sellers of these products expect the consumer to believe these claims simply by their proclamation of the existence of these plants, or special processes of obtaining CBD from other plants, instead of presenting the physical plant material for examination by peer research. Unscrupulous manufacturers and sellers may purchase CBD isolate on the wholesale market and make any claim they want to make about this stripped-down molecule since there is nothing else present.

However, there has been some valid modern research that has published about the engineering of yeast that can produce cannabinoids.[8] This is not a consumer-level product and consumers will not be able to find cannabinoids produced from yeasts as described in this research. There are no wholesale CBD isolate products available to manufacturers and retailers that are derived from yeast.

I personally recommend full-spectrum, whole-plant, lab-tested, CBD formulations, CBD-rich flowers, and raw plant products to the readers of this book. I recommend CBD products that are traceable to the farm they were grown on and purchased in state-legal dispensaries, or obtained from legal homegrown cannabis. And these full-spectrum products, because they will always contain some THC, may result in a positive drug test if you use them, even if they do not produce any psychoactive effects. Unfortunately, the drug testing industry has not yet caught up with the fact that the federal government does allow for 0.30 percent THC in hemp-derived products. CBD is not euphoric, or potentially intoxicating, although it may be somewhat sedating in higher doses. As of 2022, CBD is federally legal in the United States if it is derived from hemp.

CBCA / Cannabichromenic acid: This is one of the more commonly occurring phytocannabinoids in cannabis, but it's usually in smaller amounts than the other phytocannabinoids listed here. It is the least researched of all of the phytocannabinoids listed here. Like the other naturally occurring phytocannabinoids, it's delicate and should be extracted from a fresh flower, kept away from heat, light, oxygen, and used within about three months after extraction. CBCA is the precursor to CBC. It's almost never sold at the retail level, but it is federally legal when it is derived from hemp. It is thought to have many of the same properties as CBC, which is the more commonly available product. CBCA is not euphoric or potentially intoxicating.

---

8   Luo, X., Reiter, and L. d'Espaux. "Complete biosynthesis of cannabinoids and their unnatural analogues in yeast." *Nature* 567, 123–126 (2019). https://doi.org/10.1038/s41586-019-0978-9

CBC / Cannabichromene: As the decarboxylated product of CBCA, this phytocannabinoid has been studied for a variety of possible uses, such as use as an anti-acne medication that works by modifying oil production in skin tissue,[9] as well as a novel anti-inflammatory that works with the TRPA1 Vanilloid receptor (the same receptor that binds with capsaicin) and the CB2 (cannabinoid) receptor[10] that have been studied in human and animal models.

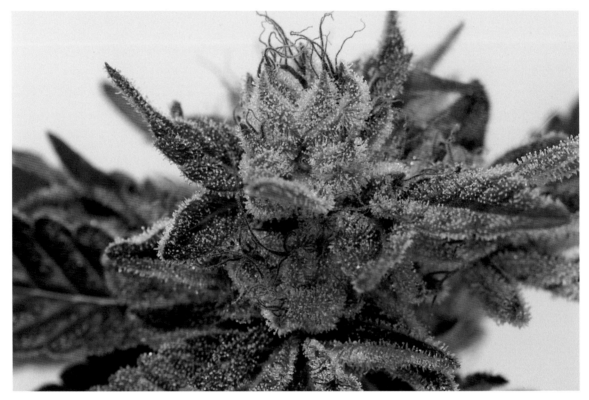

A cannabis flower with mature, milky-white, and opaque trichomes containing the phytocannabinoids and terpenes produced by the cannabis plant.

9   Oláh A. Markovics, J. Szabo. "Differential effectiveness of selected non-psychotropic phytocannabinoids on human sebocyte functions implicates their introduction in dry/seborrhoeic skin and acne treatment." *Experimental Dermatolology.* 2016 Sep; 25(9) 701.7. doi: 10.1111/exd.13042. Epub 2016 Jun 15. PMID: 27094344 https://pubmed.ncbi.nlm.nih.gov/27094344/

10 Izzo, A. A., R. Capasso, G. Aviello, F. Borrelli, B. Romano, F. Piscitelli, L. Gallo, F. Capasso, P. Orlando, and V. Di Marzo. "Inhibitory effect of cannabichromene, a major non-psychotropic cannabinoid extracted from Cannabis sativa, on inflammation-induced hypermotility in mice." *British Journal of Pharmacology.* 2012 Jun; 166(4):1444-60. doi: 10.1111/j.1476-5381.2012.01879.x. PMID: 22300105; PMCID: PMC3417459.https://pubmed.ncbi.nlm.nih.gov/22300105/

CBC is not euphoric or potentially intoxicating. As of 2022, CBC is federally legal in the United States if it is derived from hemp.

THCA / Tetrahydrocannabinolic acid: The cannabis plant produces this phytocannabinoid directly from CBGA. It is not euphoric, potentially psychedelic, or potentially intoxicating. It has many of the same benefits as THC, but without the high. Like other phytocannabinoids produced directly by the cannabis plant, it is fragile and will eventually decarboxylate into its degraded phytocannabinoid form, THC. THCA can be extracted, carefully, from fresh or freshly dried cannabis flowers. It should be used quickly once extracted to prevent the effects of THC. It stimulates the appetite, relieves pain, and has antitumor and anti-inflammatory properties.[11]

THCVA / Tetrahydrocannabivarin acid: This is produced directly by the cannabis plant like other acidic phytocannabinoids and appears in greater amounts in genetic lines originating from African sativa strains. It's common for seed sellers and dispensaries to label these if they have them because they are in great demand! THCVA has many of the same properties as its decarboxylated molecule THCV. One of the more interesting effects that is of interest is that THCVA, unlike THCA and THC, appears to have appetite control effects, which may be good for people who need to control their blood sugar.[12] THCVA is not euphoric or intoxicating.

THC / tetrahydrocannabinol / delta-9 tetrahydrocannabinol, 11-hydroxy-Δ9-tetrahydrocannabinol / THCV Tetrahydrocannabivarin / delta-8 tetrahydrocannabinol: These are the four most important Tetrahydrocannabinols. All four of these have similar effects as psychotropic cannabinoids but act in different ways.

---

11 Nallathambi, R., M. Mazuz, A. Ion, G. Selvaraj, et al., "Anti-Inflammatory Activity in Colon Models Is Derived from Δ9-Tetrahydrocannabinolic Acid That Interacts with Additional Compounds in Cannabis Extracts." *Cannabis Cannabinoid Res.* 2017 Jul 1;2(1): 167–182. doi:10.1089/can.2017.0027. PMID: 29082314; PMCID: PMC5627671. https://www.ncbi.nlm.nih.gov/pmc/articles/PMC5627671/
12 Dawson, D. A. "Synthetic Cannabinoids, Organic Cannabinoids, the Endocannabinoid System, and Their Relationship to Obesity, Diabetes, and Depression." *Mol Biol* 2018. 7: 219. doi: 10.4172/2168-9547.1000219

Synthetic and Whole-Plant Pharmaceutical THC
Euphoric, Potentially Intoxicating

The pharmaceutical THC drugs that are prescription only in the United States include the synthetic THC drugs Marinol[13] and Cesamet.[14] Doctors may write prescriptions for these drugs in any state in the United States, and they are filled by pharmacies. Sativex,[15] a whole-plant pharmaceutical drug containing both THC and CBD, is only available by prescription in Canada and Europe at this time. These products are only for use under the supervision of a licensed physician.[16] You should never operate a vehicle or any dangerous equipment while under the influence of pharmaceutical THC.

Delta-9 THC
Euphoric, Potentially Intoxicating

This is the decarboxylated molecule that comes from THCA. Delta-9 THC enters the bloodstream directly via smoking, vaping, and sometimes through mucous membranes and transdermal skin applications. Delta-9 THC is the cannabinoid most commonly associated with the "high" one will experience when using cannabis for psychoactive purposes. The effects of delta-9 THC last about two to four hours on average. Many people who use cannabis prefer delta-9 THC as a shorter-acting "high" with fewer undesirable side effects than 11 hydroxy delta-9 THC. But this is an individual matter, and each person will have a different perception of the delta-9 THC experience. Delta-9 THC is typically not psychedelic, but it can be euphoric and potentially intoxicating. Delta-9 THC does provide pain relief and appetite stimulation, as well as some of the other benefits of THCA and CBGA. You should never operate a vehicle or any dangerous equipment while under the influence of delta-9 THC.

---

13 "Marinol drug facts." FDA.gov https://www.accessdata.fda.gov/drugsatfda_docs/label/2005/018651s021lbl.pdf

14 "Cesamet drug facts." FDA.gov https://www.accessdata.fda.gov/drugsatfda_docs/label/2006/018677s011lbl.pdf

15 "Sativex drug facts." Electronic Medicines Compendium United Kingdom. https://www.medicines.org.uk/emc/product/602/smpc#gref

16 Kogan, MD, Mikhail and Joan Liebmann-Smith PhD. "Cannabis Treatment for Aches and Pains." ProjectCBD. https://www.projectcbd.org/cannabis-treatment-aches-pains

11-Hydroxy-Δ9-tetrahydrocannabinol
Euphoric, Potentially Intoxicating

This cannabinoid is only produced when the phytocannabinoid delta-9 THC passes through the gastric system and is processed in the liver to become 11-hydroxy-Δ9-tetrahydrocannabinol/11-hydroxy-THC.[17] This cannabinoid has effects that typically last six hours and can last as long as twenty-four hours, depending on how much you have ingested. Consuming anything, whether candy, brownies, oils, tinctures, or anything edible with delta-9 THC will result in the 11-hydroxy-Δ9-tetrahydrocannabinol experience. 11-hydroxy-THC is much more powerful in terms of euphoric, potentially psychedelic, or a potentially intoxicating experience. As cited in the Introduction section of this book, 11-hydroxy-THC (specifically edible cannabis products, but this compound can also form in smaller amounts after smoking cannabis)[18] is the cannabinoid that comprises the greatest number of emergency room visits for the side effects caused by overindulgence. The side effects for a beginner can be psychedelic and potentially anxiety-inducing even in moderate doses that are as little as 10 milligrams. However, in smaller doses, 11-hydroxy-THC can also be a powerful analgesic and sedative. The cannabis pharmaceuticals of a century ago were almost all oral medicines and would have had these beneficial effects. And like delta-9 THC smoked or vaporized, you should never operate a vehicle or dangerous equipment after ingesting edible products containing THC.[19]

THCV / Tetrahydrocannabivarin
Euphoric, Potentially Intoxicating

This phytocannabinoid occurs in the decarboxylation process of THCVA and has many of the same properties and effects of THCVA, including appetite control and blood-sugar

---

17 "11-hydroxy-THC." Wikipedia https://en.wikipedia.org/wiki/11-Hydroxy-THC

18 Karschner, E. L., E. W. Schwilke, R. H. Lowe, W. D. Darwin, et al., "Implications of plasma Delta9-tetrahydrocannabinol, 11-hydroxy-THC, and 11-nor-9-carboxy-THC concentrations in chronic cannabis smokers." *J Anal Toxicol*. 2009 Oct;33(8):469-77. doi: 10.1093/jat/33.8.469. PMID: 19874654; PMCID: PMC3159863. https://www.ncbi.nlm.nih.gov/pmc/articles/PMC3159863/

19 Schwilke, E. W., D. M. Schwope, and E. L. Karschner, et al. "Delta9-tetrahydrocannabinol (THC), 11-hydroxy-THC, and 11-nor-9-carboxy-THC plasma pharmacokinetics during and after continuous high-dose oral THC." *Clinical Chemistry*. 2009. 55(12):2180-2189. doi:10.1373/clinchem.2008.122119 https://academic.oup.com/clinchem/article/55/12/2180/5629430

lowering effects.[20] THCV is euphoric like THC, but milder, and many say more uplifting and energizing but without the anxiety that some users associate with THC. THCV is my favorite phytocannabinoid to chill with when I can find strains that have a lot of it! Many people, including myself, find this to be a mentally stimulating and creativity-enhancing phytocannabinoid. Like THC, you should not drive a vehicle or operate dangerous machinery while under the influence of THCV.

Delta-8 THC
Euphoric, Potentially Intoxicating

This is a phytocannabinoid occurring in trace amounts in natural cannabis resin, but it is a controversial cannabinoid as the newcomer to the cannabis scene. Because cannabis resins naturally have so little of this phytocannabinoid, it is not realistic to be able to get a meaningful amount from the resins directly. As of 2022, delta-8 THC is a gray area in federal law. Since hemp is legal, and all phytocannabinoids in hemp are legal as long as the delta-9 THC content is below 0.30 percent, delta-8 THC is technically legal, as it is produced via chemical transformation of the CBD phytocannabinoid molecule found in federally legal hemp. Delta-8 THC is an unregulated substance, and it is typically not sold in licensed and state-legal cannabis dispensaries that are subject to oversight of their products in terms of state-required regulatory testing. Delta-8 THC is primarily sold where over-the-counter CBD products are sold, that is, CBD products that come from hemp. Although no deaths have been reported from delta-8 THC, the FDA has received reports of emergency room visits due to ingesting of delta-8 THC. This seems similar to the reports that come in for visits to the emergency room due to overindulgence of the other THC phytocannabinoids.[21]

Delta-8 is purported to be a less intoxicating cannabinoid. Users do experience a mild to moderate high. And due to its current position as of 2022 as a legal gray area in many areas without legal adult-use cannabis laws and dispensaries, it has become a popular offering in retail stores and websites that sell hemp-derived CBD products.

---

20 Abioye A, O. Ayodele, A, Marinkovic, and R, Patidar et al. Δ9-Tetrahydrocannabivarin (THCV): a commentary on potential therapeutic benefit for the management of obesity and diabetes. J Cannabis Res. 2020 Jan 31;2(1):6. doi: 10.1186/s42238-020-0016-7. PMID: 33526143; PMCID: PMC7819335

21 5 Things to Know about Delta-8 Tetrahydrocannabinol—Delta-8 THC, https://www.fda.gov/consumers/consumer-updates/5-things-know-about-delta-8-tetrahydrocannabinol-delta-8-thc

Less is known about delta-8 THC than any of the other THC phytocannabinoids due to the fact that it occurs in such small amounts in natural cannabis resins and must be produced via chemical processes from CBD isolate in order to create volume for retail sale. At this time, I would not recommend this product to first-time cannabis consumers. The desirable euphoric effects you are seeking from a cannabis experience can be achieved using the naturally produced phytocannabinoid resins from the cannabis plant, which have literally thousands of years of research and human experience behind them.

But the truth is that the delta-8 THC market wouldn't even exist if it were not for the federal prohibition of cannabis plants containing THC greater than 0.30 percent. Delta-8 THC is more or less a way to circumvent the vestiges of cannabis prohibition that still remain in US federal law as of 2022. Furthermore, it's not really a plant medicine, because it requires a great deal of chemical modification of the isolated CBD molecule to produce. **In good conscience, I just can't recommend delta-8 products for anyone.**

CBN / Cannabinol: This phytocannabinoid has some of the same effects as THC and THCV and is mildly euphoric. This is the final degradation product of THC. It is primarily found in old cannabis—cannabis that has sat on a shelf for a long time or had multiple exposures to heat, light, and oxygen. Aging seems to be the greatest factor in the development of this phytocannabinoid. If you've ever smoked really old, dry cannabis flowers and noticed a foggy, sleepy feeling and not much of the same kind of "high" you normally expect from THC or THCV, it probably has CBN content. CBN is now popular in a lot of dispensary products that blend phytocannabinoids for specific purposes, such as sedatives. There is some conflicting information about the sedative effects of CBN, but anecdotally cannabis users report sedation experiences when using old/overly aged cannabis products.[22] And like THC or THCV, it's advisable not to drive a vehicle or use dangerous equipment after you have used CBN.

In addition to phytocannabinoids and other trace compounds, cannabis is rich in terpenes. *Terpenes* are the compounds that give cannabis its fragrance. Cannabis plants have the ability to produce many kinds of terpenes that produce an impressive variety of

---

22   Corroon J. "Cannabinol and Sleep: Separating Fact from Fiction." *Cannabis Cannabinoid Res.* 2021 Oct;6(5):366–371. doi: 10.1089/can.2021.0006. Epub 2021 Aug 31. PMID: 34468204; PMCID: PMC 8612407. https://pubmed.ncbi.nlm.nih.gov/34468204/

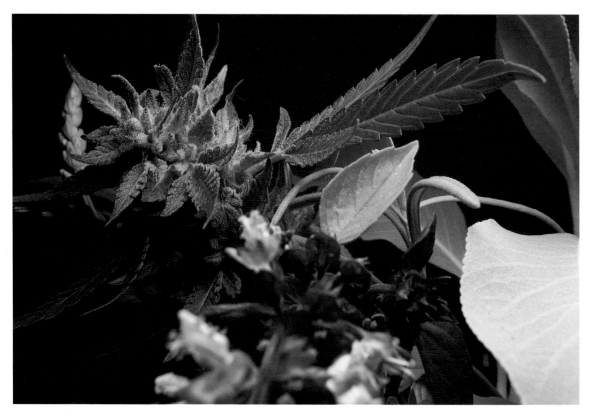

A cannabis flower bouquet, featuring herbs with many of the same terpenes found in cannabis. The fragrances of lavender, mint, basil, lemon balm, and sage are all made up of the same terpenes that occur in cannabis.

fragrances.[23] There are cannabis flowers that smell strongly of tangerines, some that are very minty, and some that smell like pine trees. There are cannabis flowers that smell like vanilla and cake, grape candy, and roses. Those are just a few of my favorite cannabis fragrances, but there are even more! All of these are possible due to the terpenes produced in the resinous trichome glands of the cannabis plant. Based on the genetics, growing methods, harvest, and curing, each of these wonderful fragrances can be produced in varying amounts, the same way phytocannabinoids are produced.

Cannabis is not a plant that stands alone and is like no other plant. It is like many other aromatic plants. If you thought that cannabis only had "that one odor," you will be pleasantly surprised to learn that cannabis produces the same terpenes that some of your other favorite

23 Sommano, S. R., C. Chittasupho, W. Ruksiriwanich, and P. Jantrawut. "The Cannabis Terpenes." *Molecules*. 2020 Dec 8;25(24):5792. doi: 10.3390/molecules25245792. PMID: 33302574; PMCID: PMC7763918. https://www.ncbi.nlm.nih.gov/pmc/articles/PMC7763918/

aromatic plants produce and that cannabis can mimic those fragrances quite well! If you are fond of essential oils, you'll be pleased to know that cannabis makes the same terpenes (fragrances) found in many of your favorite essential oil brands.

Some examples of the terpenes that occur naturally in cannabis and other aromatic plants:

- Limonene: Also in lemons and other citrus plants
- Caryophyllene: Also in black pepper and cloves
- Myrcene: Also in mangos and myrrh resin
- Linalool: Also in lavender and agastache
- Pinene: Also in pine needles and rosemary
- Geraniol: Also in roses and geranium (pelargonium)

The Entourage Effect

About a decade ago, Dr. Sanjay Gupta hosted a news documentary special on CNN about CBD and introduced the concept of the "entourage effect" to the mainstream public. Many

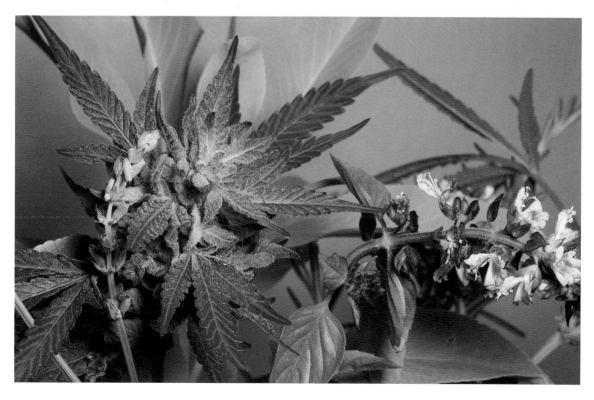

people had never heard of CBD, let alone the fact that all of the compounds in cannabis, including all of the cannabinoids and terpenes, worked together as an "entourage" that was much more effective than any cannabinoid stripped down alone.

We can't talk about cannabinoids and the entourage effect without talking about the system in our body that is designed specifically for cannabinoids to bind themselves to—the endocannabinoid system.[24] Indeed, the human body makes an endocannabinoid called *anandamide*. This cannabinoid is called an endocannabinoid because it is made and processed inside our bodies. Anandamide binds to our CB1 and CB2 receptors and interacts with the vanilloid receptor.[25] The vanilloid receptor is also activated by capsaicin, the compound in chili peppers that makes them hot.[26] The phytocannabinoids naturally produced by cannabis, and the phytocannabinoids that are the product of decarboxylation, also bind to the receptors of our endocannabinoid system. The endocannabinoid system plays an important role in a wide variety of bodily functions, which explains to a great degree the variety and versatility of phytocannabinoid medicine. Throughout history, cannabis has been employed for the purpose of treating a wide variety of symptoms and conditions.[27]

The differences between full-spectrum and stripped-down cannabinoids are noticeable, and the effects or lack of effect are disappointing in stripped-down cannabinoid products. In a pinch, in a location where only a stripped-down molecule is legal, like CBD-only products, or in a situation involving drug testing for the presence of THC, it's possible to build an entourage around a CBD-only product, with the addition of terpenes from other aromatics and the addition of other herbs. I describe these techniques in my book *CBD and Hemp Remedies* for those who only have access to CBD-only oils and other products—but it's not going to be as effective or satisfying as using a full-spectrum cannabis product. It's not possible for a skilled chemist to duplicate the entourage effect contained in a full spectrum cannabis extract; and it's certainly not possible for the home or spa herbalist to duplicate the more than four hundred compounds in cannabis that make up the entourage effect.

---

24 "Endocannabinoid System." ScienceDirect.com. https://www.sciencedirect.com/topics/pharmacology
   -toxicology-and-pharmaceutical-science/endocannabinoid-system
25 "Endocannabinoids." ScienceDirect.com. https://www.sciencedirect.com/topics/pharmacology-toxicology-and
   -pharmaceutical-science/endocannabinoids
26 "Vanilloid Receptor." ScienceDirect.com. https://www.sciencedirect.com/topics/medicine-and-dentistry
   /vanilloid-receptor
27 "Cannabinoids." Science Direct.com. https://www.sciencedirect.com/topics/pharmacology-toxicology-and
   -pharmaceutical-science/cannabinoids

It's important to remember that modern cannabinoid research is an emerging field in science—there is still so much more to learn. I always advise "medical cannabis" patients who are newly minted medical cannabis cardholders to speak with a licensed medical doctor with experience serving medical cannabis patients before attempting to treat any condition with cannabis to ensure good outcomes. This could be the doctor who wrote your medical card recommendation or another doctor who specializes in medicinal cannabis medicine specifically. This is a valuable resource for ensuring that all your current conditions, medications, and treatments are compatible with the medicinal use of cannabis.

Cannabis Plant Products

This list of cannabis plant products represents what most people will encounter at legal dispensaries or when growing at home. When crafting your first-time experience, think about which products of the cannabis plant will be ideal for your individual experience and make a mental note of these for the mindfulness exercise in the next section.

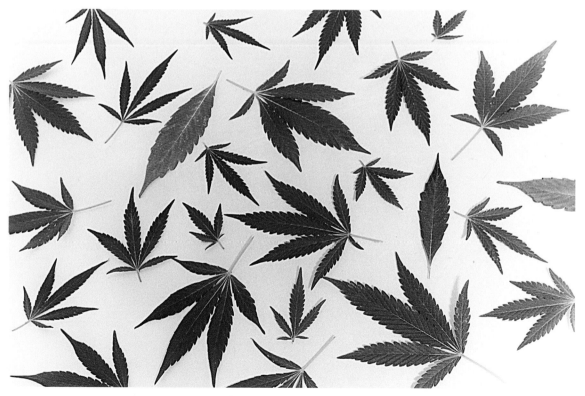

Various shapes and sizes of cannabis fan leaves.

Leaves, specifically the fan leaf of the cannabis plant, is a temperate green vegetable that contains no or few phytocannabinoids and is typically used in recipes calling for bitter greens or any recipe that works well with bitter greens. They can also be used as culinary or spa garnishes.

Seeds of the cannabis plant have high levels of complete proteins and have high amounts of Omega-3 and fiber. They are free of all phytocannabinoids. They are excellent for making smoothies and for all kinds of culinary uses. You can also grow new cannabis plants with them.

Stems of the cannabis plant are sometimes used in flavoring soups and sauces in Thai cuisine. These have use, as the roots do, in imparting that coveted umami flavor in Asian cuisine.[28] Depending on the variety of cannabis used, stems may also contain higher levels of sticky

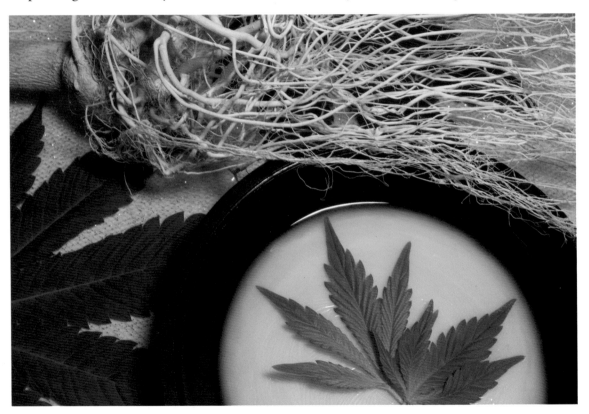

Roots and leaves of the cannabis plant.

28 "Amid narcotics reform, Thai cooks replace MSG with cannabis." TheWorld.org. April 21, https://the world.org/stories/2021-04-23/amid-narcotics-reform-thai-cooks-replace-msg-cannabis

phytocannabinoid resin—so for any edible application where you desire a nonpsychoactive experience, it is advisable to use the hemp varieties of cannabis low in potential THC.

Roots of the cannabis plant have an ancient history as a medicament for both internal and external use. While they don't contain phytocannabinoids, they do contain other compounds, like phytosterols and compounds unique to the cannabis plant like cannabisativine. These compounds have anti-inflammatory and antiseptic properties. Some of the traditional uses of the cannabis root include boiling the root and using it as a kind of poultice for tumors.[29]

This is very similar to the Appalachian herbalist method of using poke root (Phytolacca *americana*) as a boiled poultice for tumor and inflammation relief. In fact, many of the traditional uses of cannabis root appear to be practically identical to the ways that poke root has been deployed in Appalachian folk medicine—a practice I am personally familiar with through my own family lore. But unlike poke root, cannabis root is not toxic. Poke root requires a skilled hand and many years of herbal studies due to the potential for toxin exposure. Even then, the possible danger of poke root for the average person working with herbs is too great for me to recommend the root of Phytolacca *americana* as an herb to practice with.

Cannabis roots are safe to work with, are nonpsychoactive, and can be prepared as poultices, salves, and decoctions.

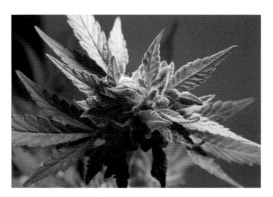

The mature and very resinous cannabis flower can be used for many purposes.

Pollen only occurs in the male flowers of male or hermaphrodite cannabis plants. It is sometimes kept dry and in cold storage for plant-breeding programs.

Female flowers are the most popular plant product of the cannabis plant. They are a versatile way to use the naturally occurring phytocannabinoids in cannabis. The whole flowers contain the intact naturally occurring terpenes, phytocannabinoids,

29 Ryz, N. R., D. J. Remillard, and E. B. Russo. "Cannabis Roots: A Traditional Therapy with Future Potential for Treating Inflammation and Pain." *Cannabis Cannabinoid Res.* 2017; 2(1):210-216. Published 2017 Aug 1. doi:10.1089/can.2017.0028 https://www.liebertpub.com/doi/10.1089/can.2017.0028

and other trace compounds. They can be vaporized, smoked, made into oil and tinctures, or used whole in edible or topical and transdermal preparations.

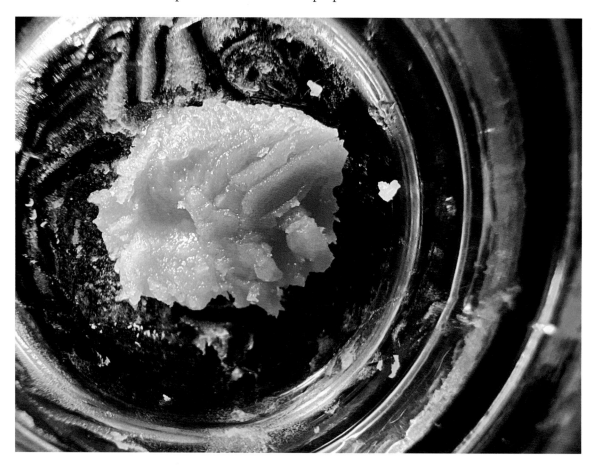

Live rosin is a petroleum-free, concentrated phytocannabinoid and terpene resin derived from cannabis flowers. It contains the highest amount of terpenes of any of the other phytocannabinoid concentrates listed here. Live rosin is produced by subjecting fresh cannabis flowers to a great deal of pressure and literally squeezing the resin out of them. This is a highly concentrated product that is not recommended for first-time or novice cannabis users. This product is not recommended for a first-time cannabis experience due to the attentiveness and knowledge required to serve accurate dosages of this highly concentrated product.

Kif is the trichomes of the dried and cured cannabis flower that have been shaken or sifted from the whole flowers. It is less concentrated than live rosin and many oil extracts but has about the same amount of phytocannabinoid content as hashish. It retains quite a bit of the natural terpene content, more than hashish or oil extracts as the trichomes are mostly intact. This product is okay for novices but not suggested for a first timer. It's more concentrated than whole flowers, and a new user must be cautious not to use as much kif as flower when vaping, smoking, or using in an edible product.

Hashish is the concentrated trichome content of the cannabis flower and is produced by several methods. Traditional Moroccan and Indian methods of production include rolling the cannabis flowers in the hand so that the sticky resins are removed from the flowers and can be rolled into long strings or balls. Hashish can also be made through an ice water extraction process that produces a fairly high-quality product depending on the quality of the cannabis being used.

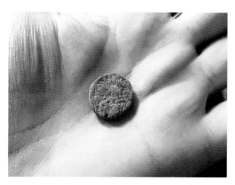

A pressed cake of ice water hashish.

Hashish, unlike kif, is a solid and sometimes hard substance that can be broken into pieces and smoked, vaporized, or used in edibles or topicals. It retains some of the naturally occurring terpenes in cannabis but not as much as live rosin and kif.

Oil extract include cannabis resin extractions using culinary-grade ethyl alcohol. Sometimes the thick oil extract made by processing with alcohol is called "full-extract cannabis oil" or alternatively "Rick Simpson oil," after the name of the man who popularized this oil in medicinal cannabis applications. It is typically not a product that can be vaped or smoked, but it can be used in edibles or topicals.

Strain Selection

This list is a basic guide to the cannabis strains you will encounter. There are always variations in what your individual experience will be with any particular strain. Keeping a strain notebook is a great way to try different strains and review your experiences!

Sativa strains: These tend to be tropical and the strains of warm geography: African, Thailand, South America. They are tall plants with slender leaves. Sativa strains also dominate the European hemp varieties high in CBD and CBG. They can be more energizing in their effects, but this is not necessarily true for all of them.

Indica strains: These are shorter, bushier plants with wide leaves. They occur in locations such as Afghanistan, India, and North Africa/Middle East. These are the cannabis plants encountered by Dr. O'Shaughnessy in the nineteenth century and the strain used to manufacture the cannabis pharmaceutical medicines of the period. Indica strains have many of the medicinal effects sought out by medical cannabis patients, including pain relief, spasm relief, and as a sedative.

Hybrid strains: These strains are created by cannabis farmers by combining the best traits of the landrace strains originating as either sativa or indica. They are a blend of these genetics and have effects that reflect the blending of these genetics. Leaves and height have attributes of both sativa and indica. Most modern strains you will encounter are hybrid strains.

Your First Plant

Growing cannabis is a botanical art that has great masters much like the art of painting has its great masters.

Because of this, growing cannabis can seem overwhelming for a beginner. If you've ever browsed any popular cannabis magazine publications, or scrolled through #cannabis on

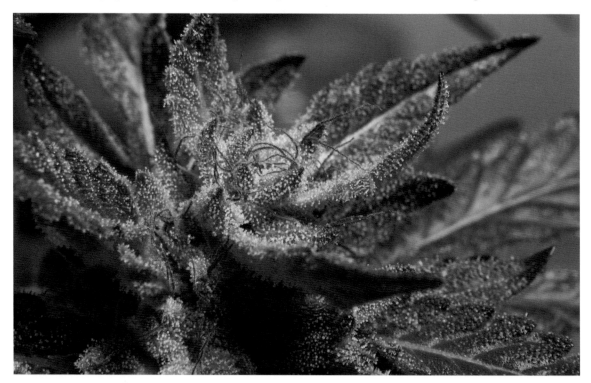

Instagram, you have been enraptured by the beauty of these plants grown by the masters of this botanical art and the final product they produce. You may also feel overwhelmed if you've ever browsed a retail store specializing in cannabis growing equipment based on the sheer magnitude of various growing apparatus, luxury fertilizers, and extensive lighting systems for indoor grows. All of this just to grow something that I'm going to like, or something that will help me feel better? Overwhelming indeed.

When I grew my first cannabis plant in 2013, I wasn't expecting much. It was a hilarious experiment, because I didn't expect much to come out of that little clone of "LA Confidential" that I had purchased at the dispensary after a budtender persuaded me to purchase one with the assurance that I would get something I liked out of it.

I had a simple two-gallon clay pot and a bag of soil that was recommended for cannabis growing by the garden store clerk. I grew this little clone indoors in a very sunny spot. When the day came that I wanted it to start making flowers, I would manually move it in and out of a dark hall closet and back into the bright, sunny area for twelve hours each day. Pretty soon I started seeing female flowers beginning to grow. And by the end of about two months of going back and forth from the dark closet into the light for twelve hours every day, I had flowers ready to harvest. About a half of an ounce (14 grams). I manicured the little flowers, hung them up to dry, and then cured them in an amber glass jar for a short cure of about two weeks. I was ready for the taste test.

I ground up some cured flower and loaded it into my tabletop vaporizer. It didn't take long before I knew that I wouldn't be driving the car for the rest of the day. Success! Okay, so it wasn't the Rolls-Royce Dispensary Top-Shelf Mega-Flower, but the flowers looked good, smelled good, tasted good, and more importantly, I now had a half of an ounce of mid-grade (15 percent THC, or thereabouts) cured cannabis flowers for the cost of the bag of soil ($10) and the little clone I bought from the dispensary ($10).

Because I had a very good cannabis strain and had met most of the plant's growing requirements, I ended up with a profit (so to speak) on my investment based on the current market value of mid-grade cannabis flowers at my local dispensary in 2013.

I discovered that cannabis really does grow like a weed, and it really only needs a few things to grow the kind of flowers that will be worth the time and investment you put into it. As a beginner, it's not necessary to spend much to grow a small harvest of 7 to 14 grams.

Today, I own a lot more growing equipment and accessories, and of course I use fertilizers to maximize my harvests. I grow indoors and outdoors, depending on the season. Over the years,

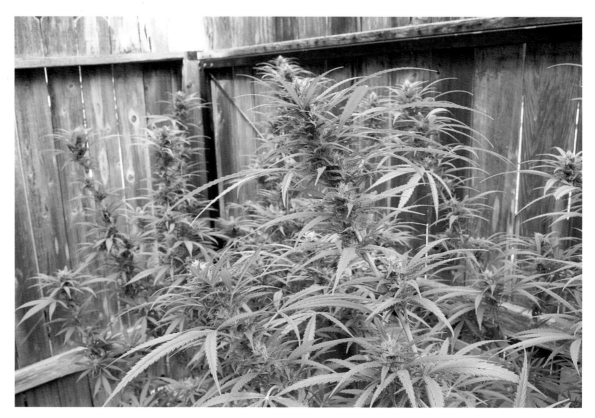

I've grown some very lovely flowers. My beginner's experience with one plant gave me the confidence to take it a bit further and buy the tent, the lights, the fertilizers, the grow books written by the masters, and dive into growing the maximum number of plants allowed by law in my state.

In this section, you are going to learn to grow your first plant for the purposes of gaining some self-confidence, one that will result in a small first-time harvest but without the commitment and effort required for larger harvests. I think that for a beginner, starting with a simple one-plant grow to get a feel for what is actually possible is the best first step—the opportunity to discover the botany of cannabis in a hands-on way.

This section is by no means comprehensive. In the Resources section of this book, you will find book titles from the masters of the art of cannabis botany, so that in the future, if you decide you would like to pursue cannabis growing, you will have resources for more extensive education on the subject.

Remember that even if you are in a location where cannabis is legal, there may be additional regulations for growing cannabis. Always ensure that you are in compliance with all laws and regulations before you grow your first plant.

Grow Setup for One Plant

Cannabis has three stages of growth: vegetation (very leafy, no flowers), flowering (all the flowering stages up to the point of harvest), and harvest (trichomes showing a milky as opposed to a clear appearance interspersed with some trichomes that appear amber in color, along with orange-ish stigmas that are white or pinkish when the flowers are immature). The equipment you will need for all three stages of cannabis growth:

One- to two-gallon felt grow bag: These are inexpensive and can be found online or in many gardening stores. The advantage of the felt grow bag over something like a clay or resin pot is that, being lightweight, they are superior for keeping the roots of the plant pruned and healthy. A one-gallon pot is going to grow a smaller plant and a smaller harvest than a two-gallon pot.

High-quality soil: This is the most important item on this list. To grow a plant that is going to give you usable flowers, do not buy cheap soil, but you can buy the smallest bag of high-quality soil to fill your pot. Some soil brands are popular with cannabis growers and some have been developed for cannabis growing. These soils will have all the basic nutrients for the short vegetation stage you will be taking the plant through. Your first plant will have a very short vegetation period before you take it to the flowering stage.

One of the most common problems with cannabis plants is nutrient deficiency of minerals like calcium, magnesium, copper, iron, etc. Starting with the highest-quality potting soil designed for growing cannabis is the best defense against these problems.

Blackstrap molasses: You may already have this item in your kitchen cabinet, but in the instance that you don't, you will want to purchase a small bottle of this to use with your first plant.

This item will be used primarily when you water your flowering cannabis plant, and it is sufficient in providing the right nutrients for a small flowering cannabis plant.

I have also used blackstrap molasses to correct nutrient deficiency. If you notice your vegetation-stage plant has curling or yellow leaves, you can water with blackstrap molasses to correct many of the most common nutrient deficiencies. As a general rule, though, if you used good-quality soil during a short vegetation stage for a small plant between 6 and 9 inches tall, you probably won't need to correct any nutrient deficiencies.

Trimming scissors for pruning: Buy an inexpensive pair of trim/pruning scissors at your local garden store. You will need these for not only the trimming of your harvest, but also for pruning the plant during growth and flower cycles. Always clean your scissors with alcohol to sanitize before pruning your plant.

Jeweler's loupe or magnifying glass to view trichomes: You are going to need magnification to check the progress of the trichomes from clear to milky and amber when the flowers are ready for harvest. It's also a great idea to own a jeweler's loupe for your trips to the dispensary so that you can examine flowers and concentrates before you purchase them.

A totally dark closet or a cardboard box covered with a black or dark cloth: During the flowering stage, you will need to make sure that your plant is not exposed to any light for twelve hours a day. This can be accomplished by placing your plant in a totally dark closet for twelve hours like I did when I grew my first plant, or covering your plant with a cardboard box covered with a black or dark cloth to block out all light.

80 percent or higher isopropyl or ethyl alcohol: You will need one bottle of this to clean your trim scissors and hands while you grow your first plant.

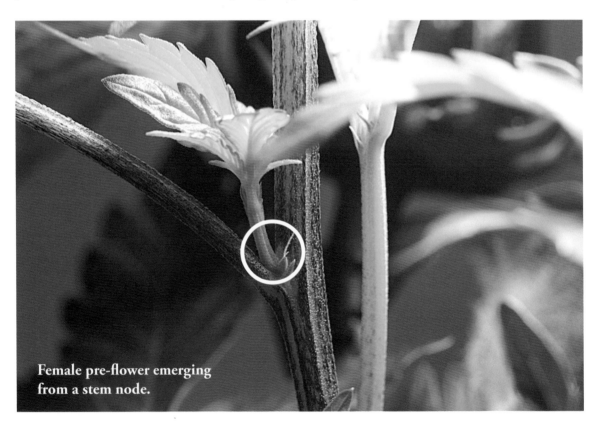

Female pre-flower emerging from a stem node.

A sunny enclosed patio or backyard, or an area in your home that gets at least eight to twelve hours of direct sunlight and at least four hours or more of indirect sunlight: For your vegetation stage to work correctly, you will want to time your grow during the spring and summer seasons that have more than fourteen hours of light per day. To compensate, you can get a small, freestanding grow light to give your plant additional hours of light up to sixteen hours per day if you want to grow during the darker seasons of winter or fall.

Feminized Seed or Clone?

You will want to grow your first plant either from a feminized seed (seed bred specifically to only grow a female plant) or a clone. Clones can be bought from the dispensary in most legal areas, or they can be taken from a friend's vegetation-stage cannabis plant.

To grow a sprout from a feminized seed you will need six items:

- a small cup
- hydrogen peroxide
- paper towels
- a shallow dish
- a spoon and measuring spoon
- tweezers

1. In the small cup, fill with 1 tablespoon (15 ml) hydrogen peroxide and 3 tablespoons (45 ml) of tepid warm water. Put your seed in the cup and push it down into the water to make sure it gets wet. If it floats, that's okay. Leave it in this water for about 4 hours.
2. Afterward, take a paper towel and fold it into quarters. It should be square with two layers of paper towel, top and bottom.
3. Remove the seed from the water cup and use the paper towel to soak up water from the cup. Place the paper towel on the shallow dish and moisten it again with another batch of the water and hydrogen peroxide mixture from the first step. It should be very moist.
4. Place the seed inside the paper towel and set the dish in a warm area. I like to pop my seeds on top of my refrigerator near the back where it is warm and dark.
5. Check every day that there is sufficient moisture in the towel and to see if a root has appeared. Typically, I let it remain in the paper towel until the second day after I have seen the root emerge from the seed.

6. The little sprout is now ready to plant. Make a hole about as deep as the first knuckle on your finger. Do not pick up the sprout with your fingers! Use a tweezer or a spoon to carefully scoop it up and drop the seed into the hole and cover it lightly with soil. Don't press down. Moisten the soil with water. In about 3 to 7 days, the seedling will emerge if you have followed these steps carefully and if your seed was viable. Keep it moist like a wrung-out sponge but not soggy. Overwatering is the number one reason a seedling will die!

Taking a clone from a vegetation-stage cannabis plant is just as easy:

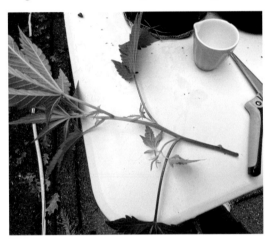

This cut should be a sturdy branch from the mother plant. Cut the stem an inch below one of the nodes.

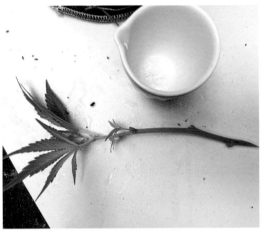

Remove all of the bottom and midsection leaves and manicure the top leaves to maximize water retention in the clone until it roots.

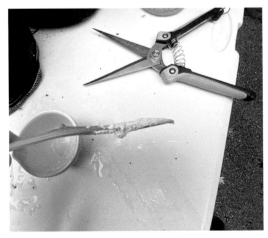

Dip the stem in rooting hormone up to the node.

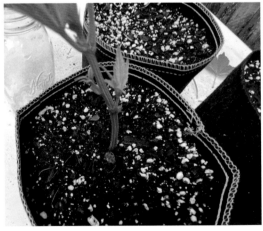

Use your finger or a stick to make a hole deep enough to cover the tip of rooting hormone and put in the cut stem. That's it!

Keep the soil about as moist as a wrung-out sponge but not soggy. You may notice that your cutting becomes a bit droopy—typically this is okay and it will revive itself if the soil is kept moist and the cutting is kept in indirect sunlight until it has a chance to form roots and you begin to see it revive with some new leaves starting to form. At this point it may be moved into the direct sun. This process may take seven to ten days. Alternatively, you can purchase clones at many legal dispensaries. This is a great option because they are already rooted and ready to begin their vegetation stage in your pot.

All the Steps for Your One-Plant Grow

After you have followed the steps with your choice of feminized seed or clone, you are ready to start the vegetation stage.

1. Place your seedling or clone on a sunny porch or a sunny area in your home. Leave this plant uncovered and allow it to absorb all the natural light as instructed above. As long as the area you have placed your plant in has some nighttime darkness (like an outdoor grow), this will be sufficient to take you through the vegetation stage. A vegetation-stage cannabis plant needs to be exposed to some light for at least 14 to 16 hours a day. This can be a mix of mostly direct light and some indirect light. Anything less than this will start the flowering cycle too early.

2. Depending on the size of pot you have chosen, this will determine the time in vegetation. Generally speaking, a 1-gallon (4.5 L) pot should be allowed to remain in the vegetation state until it reaches about 6 inches (153 mm) in height and is lush and full of leaves. A plant in a 2-gallon (9 L) pot can remain in the vegetation stage until it is about 9 inches (229 mm) and is lush and full of leaves. Depending on the strain you are growing, and whether it is a seed or a clone, this could take anywhere from 2 to 4 weeks, but no more than that. You don't want your plant to get too big for the 1- or 2-gallon pot you are using in order to conserve as much soil nutrients as possible.

3. Watering is necessary when the soil becomes dry to the touch one finger knuckle deep. If it feels dry and the pot feels light, it's time to water. Always keep your pot in a big plant dish of some type and water from the bottom. **Watering from the bottom prevents fungus gnats, which can spread fungal disease from the soil to the upper parts of the**

plant. Tap water that has sat overnight in the open air is suggested for your plant, as tap water also contains some minerals useful to the plant, unlike distilled or filtered water.

4. As mentioned earlier, if you purchased high-quality soil, nutrient deficiency should not be an issue for this size of plant. But if you notice that your leaves are yellowing during the vegetation stage, or curling, give in a good watering with 1 tablespoon (15 ml) of blackstrap molasses mixed into some tepid warm water.

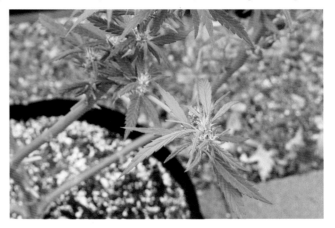

5. The vegetation stage is the perfect time to harvest a few leaves and try them out in nonpsychoactive culinary creations! Don't harvest too many and wait until the plant is at least 9 inches (229 mm) tall if you want to harvest a few leaves. I don't suggest leaf harvesting like this for smaller vegetation. If you find that you really enjoy what cannabis has to offer as a nonpsychoactive vegetable, you could grow plants of any sex (bunk seed that comes from low-quality buds is fine for this purpose) to the vegetation stage and harvest them just for their green leaves. You'll find some of these nonpsychoactive recipe suggestions in chapter 6.

Get ready to flower! Once your vegetation-stage plants are lush and at the desired height, it's time to start the flowering cycle!

1. Prepare either a dark closet or the cardboard box covered with a black or dark cloth to prevent light leaks. If you choose to use cardboard, you may need to use two or more boxes to build enough height to accommodate your flowering plant, which will double in height or a little more during the flowering stage.

2. For the flowering stage to be successful, your plant must spend 12 hours in darkness, every day, for 8 to 10 weeks, no exceptions. Try to remain on schedule with this as much as possible, because too much variation or forgetfulness can send the plant into a hermaphrodite stage, which you do not want. Twelve hours every day in total darkness is required for healthy flowers.

3. Trim the bottom leaves and branches, leaving a space of at least 2 inches between leaves and branches and the soil. This will ensure good air circulation. Plants in the flowering

stage need good air circulation especially if you are in a humid environment (but, really, in every environment). Flowers can be quite lush and subject to developing mold if there is not enough air circulation. A fan to circulate the air for at least 4 hours a day or an open window to allow for circulation near your plant will be sufficient.

4. Use the touch method to determine the watering schedule. If the soil is dry down to the first knuckle on your finger and the pot seems light, it's time to water. Don't wait for a wilted plant to water it because this is the kind of stress that can bring out hermaphrodite characteristics.

5. You will likely be watering now twice a week or a little more. You need to water once a week with a mixture of 1 tablespoon (15 ml) of blackstrap molasses mixed into tepid warm water. As during the vegetation stage, tap water is suggested for additional minerals. Continue to water from the bottom to prevent fungus gnats. If, during the flowering stage, you notice any of these little gnats, you can place a small sticky trap on top of the soil to control them. Use a plain soapy spray on top of the soil if they continue to be a problem.

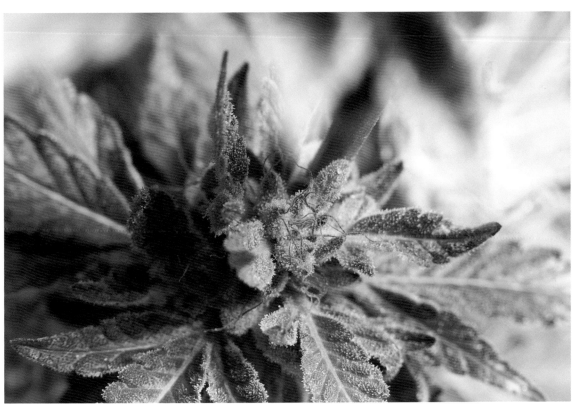

6. Note the white or pinkish female flower stigmas and the clear trichomes forming on your plant. These will look much different during the harvesting cycle.

7. Your plant will remain in the flowering stage for 8 to 10 weeks as a general rule of thumb with 12 hours of total darkness and 12 hours of mostly direct and some indirect light every day.

8. You will begin to notice during the latter part of the flowering stage that fan leaves are starting to yellow or change color. This is natural and not a nutrient deficiency. Simply trim these leaves using clean trimming scissors.

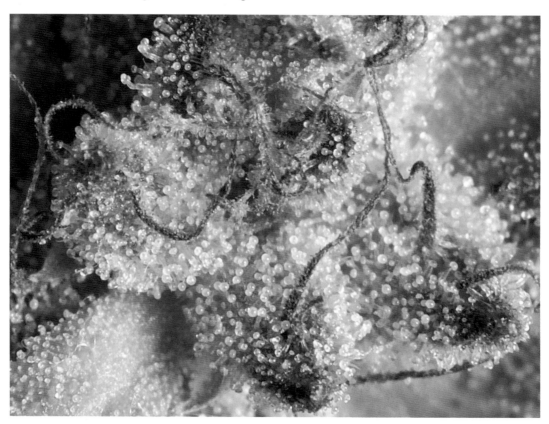

When and How to Harvest

1. When your flowers are ready for harvest, the trichomes will be milky, as opposed to clear, with some of the trichomes taking on an amber hue. The stigmas will be orange or reddish and look dry. This is the peak moment your plant is ready for harvest!

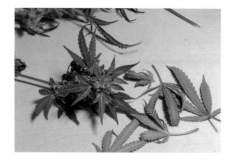

2. Before harvesting, flush your plant thoroughly with lots of clean water (no molasses) for 3 days before harvesting. Don't worry about overwatering at this point. The flush is good for the plant to take up water without any nutrients right before harvest.

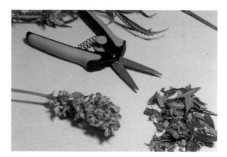

3. First, cut all of the stems down to the last two inches before the root. Next, use your trim scissors to remove all of the fan leaves as seen in the photo.

4. Now it's time to trim those sugar leaves! These are the leaves that grow out of the flower bracts and typically have trichomes. You will want to set these aside and let them dry to use in edible or topical recipes, or to make a cannabis oil.

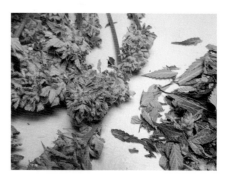

5. After all of your flowers have been trimmed and you have separated the sugar leaf into another pile, tie up all of the trimmed flowers on their stems and hang them upside down in an area that is dry but does not get any sunlight. Sunlight will degrade the cannabinoids and terpenes. It's a good idea to have lots of good air circulation around them while they dry. If necessary, use a fan to circulate the air while they dry. Depending on your environment, your flowers should be dry enough to cure within a week.

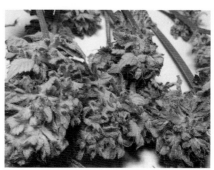

Curing Your Harvest

After your flowers are dry, it's time to cure them. You will know that the flowers are dry enough to cure when the stems readily snap and break instead of bending. Take them down from where they were hanging to dry and use your trimming scissors to cut the flower buds from the stems. Put the flowers into an amber or other dark glass or ceramic jar. Keep in mind that there may still be some moisture in the flowers, so you don't want to seal them up in the jar for more than a day or two. Then gently shake the jar and open it to air out for a day. Close the jar again and repeat this step until the flowers are not moist. Most flowers have sufficiently cured for my taste after about three weeks. Some people prefer longer or shorter cures. During this time, they will also lose chlorophyll. This is good, because the flowers will make for a smoother smoke or vaping experience. If your flowers seem a little "harsh" when you vaporize or smoke them, just allow them to cure in the jar for a little longer.

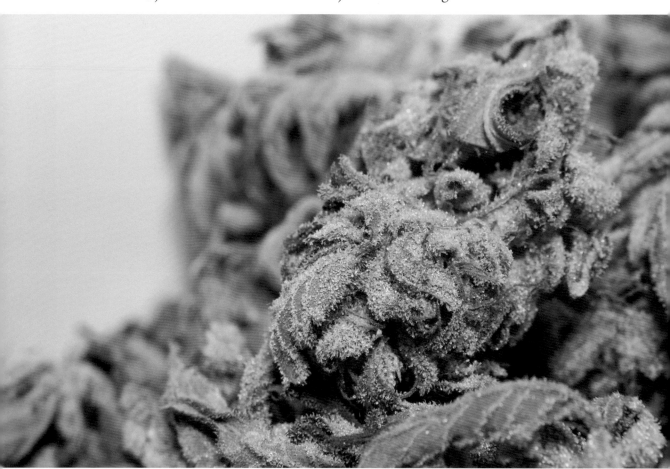

Cannabis as a Vegetable: Easy, Nonpsychoactive Recipes and Techniques for First-Time Growers

Did you know that the fan leaves of the cannabis plant are a delicious and nonpsychoactive green vegetable? Fan leaves often go into the compost pile or trash during the growing process when they should really be on your dinner menu! I have included my two favorite recipes using cannabis fan leaves here. If you are growing cannabis for the first time, take advantage of everything this incredible plant has to offer—the fan leaves should never go to waste when you can add them to green smoothies or prepare them in my two favorite fan-leaf recipes.

Selecting and preparing fan leaves for consumption:

Select healthy green cannabis fan leaves. If they are a little faded, or slightly yellowed, this is okay. Don't use leaves that are brown and all yellow or any leaf that is compromised with disease. Cut away all of the "finger" of the leaf to use in these recipes and toss the more fibrous part of the leaf they are attached to.

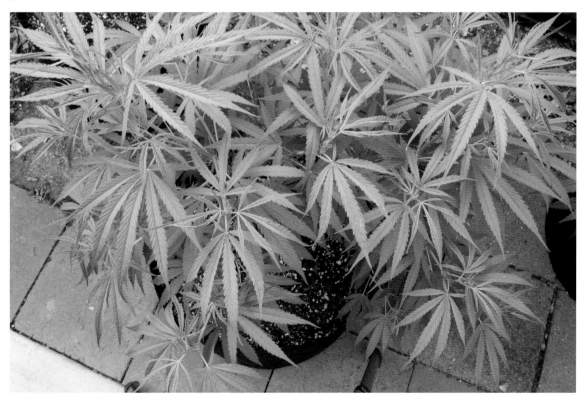

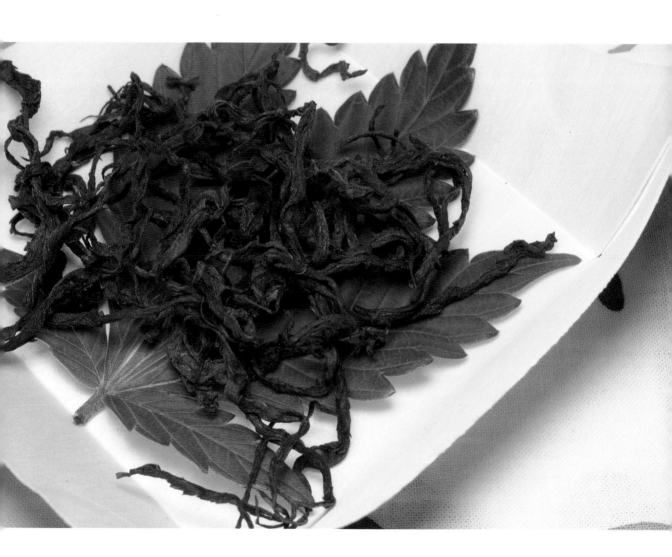

Naoko's Japanese Cannabis Leaf Condiment

This Japanese-style condiment was introduced to me by my friend from Japan. Cannabis isn't legal in Japan, so she makes this at her home here in the States. In Japan, there are all kinds of toppings for rice, and these are called "friends of rice." This recipe is just that: it's a friend of rice, but it's also chewy, crunchy, umami, a little sweet, and spicy too, at least that's how I make it. This is my favorite remix of her cannabis leaf condiment. And it's vegan!

Serving size depends on size of leaves

Ingredients:
30 large cannabis fan leaves, main leaf stem removed from leaf fingers
1 tablespoon (15 ml) mirin
2 teaspoons (10 ml) tamari
2 teaspoons (10 ml) ginger juice
1 teaspoon (3 g) sugar
Optional: 1 fresh hot pepper or less depending on your heat tolerance, finely chopped
2 teaspoons (10 ml) toasted sesame oil

Instructions:

1. After you have rinsed and cut the cannabis leaf fingers away from the main leaf stem, pat them dry and put them in a bowl.

2. Add the mirin, tamari, and ginger. Massage these ingredients into the cannabis leaves. Let them marinate in this mixture covered and on the counter for 6 hours. Stir occasionally to distribute liquid evenly.

3. The mixture may have a bit more liquid than what you started with after the leaves wilt and marinate. Strain off this excess liquid and stir in the sugar, optional hot pepper, and sesame oil to thoroughly coat all the leaves.

4. Spread the leaves out on a dehydrator pan, and dehydrate on the warm setting. Alternatively, you may dehydrate in the oven by spreading the leaves out on a baking sheet lined with parchment paper. Set the oven at the lowest temperature and put the tray in and crack the oven door just a little.

5. The condiment is ready when the leaves are dehydrated, chewy with some crispiness. These are shelf-stable if kept in a container with a moisture absorbing pack.

6. Enjoy these right out of the container, or put them on vegetables, rice, or soup.

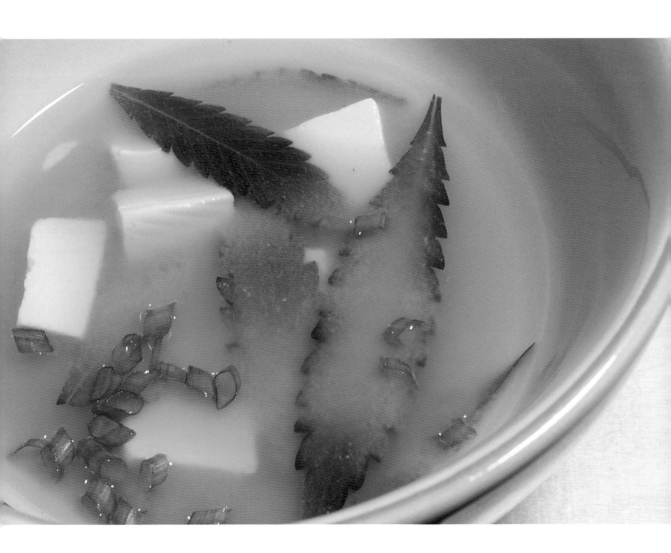

Cannabis Leaf Miso Soup

I came up with this recipe one day when I ran out of nori sheets to slice for miso soup. No nori but plenty of cannabis fan leaves, so I just went with it! It turned out great, and now I always use cannabis leaves in place of nori. Both kombu and cannabis stalk infuse additional umami flavor into this vegan soup.

Makes approximately 4 servings

Ingredients:

1 quart + 1 cup of water (1 liter + 240 ml)
1 piece kombu
1 cannabis stalk (the thicker main stem of the plant) the same size (6 inches (15 cm))
1 tablespoon (15 ml) mirin
¼ cup (60 ml) white miso paste (a little more or less, adjust for your own taste)
Optional: grated fresh ginger to taste
½ pound (0.25 kilo) tofu, drained and cubed
10 large cannabis fan leaves, main leaf stem removed from leaf fingers
chopped spring onion, for garnish

Instructions:

1. Make dashi first. Add the water, kombu, cannabis stalk, and mirin to a pan on the stove. Cover and simmer gently on medium-low for 45 minutes. Turn off the stove and allow the dashi to cool, covered, for about 30 more minutes. Remove the kombu and cannabis stalk.

2. Return the pan to the stove and turn the heat back on. Add the miso paste and stir. Bring this to a lively simmer and add the optional grated ginger and the tofu. Simmer for 3 minutes.

3. Add the fresh cannabis fan leaves and simmer for 3 more minutes. Remove from the stove.

4. Stir briskly and ladle into bowls. Sprinkle spring onion on top. Optionally you may also sprinkle some sesame seeds and/or cannabis leaf condiment. Serve immediately.

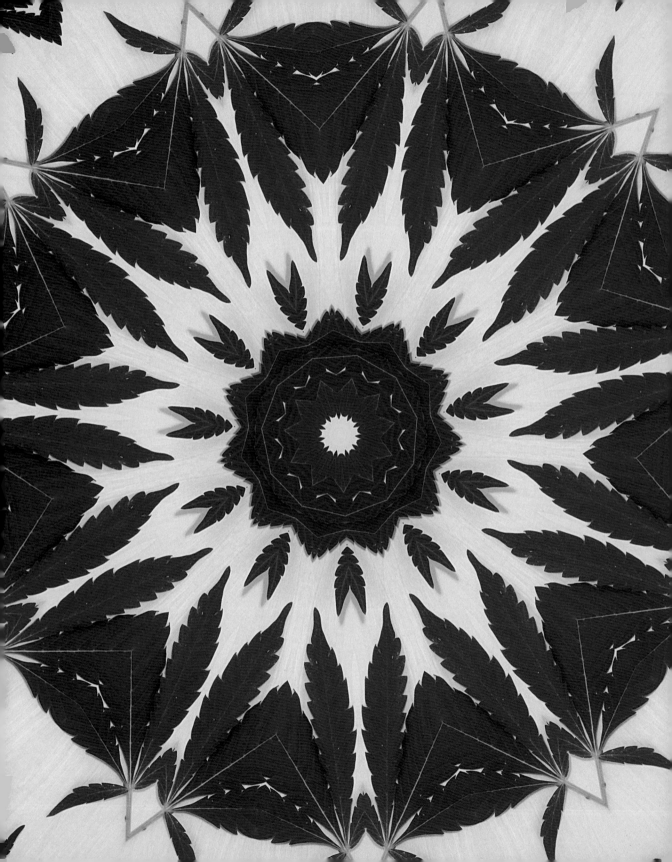

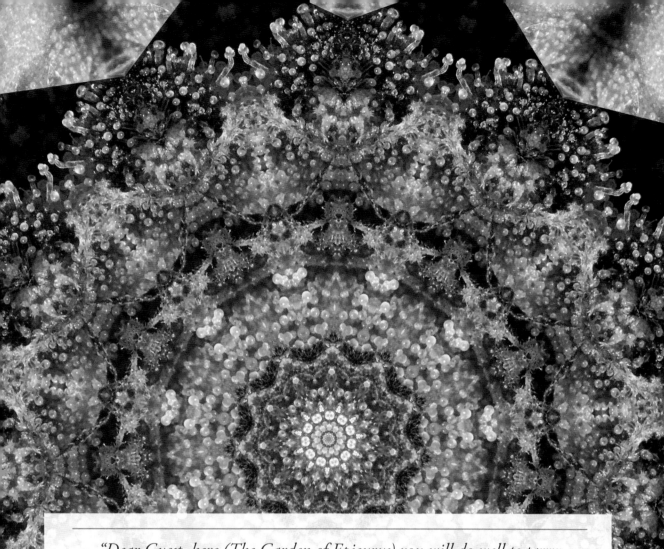

"*Dear Guest, here (The Garden of Epicurus) you will do well to tarry; here our highest good is pleasure.*" The caretaker of that abode, a friendly host, will be ready for you; he will welcome you with barley-meal, and serve you water also in abundance, with these words: "*Have you not been well entertained? This garden does not whet your appetite; but quenches it. Nor does it make you more thirsty with every drink; it slakes the thirst with a natural cure—a cure that requires no fee. It is with this type of pleasure that I have grown old.*"
Seneca—*Letters to Lucilius (21.10)*[30]

30 Seneca—*Letters to Lucilius (21.10)* http://wiki.epicurism.info/Epicurus%27_Garden/

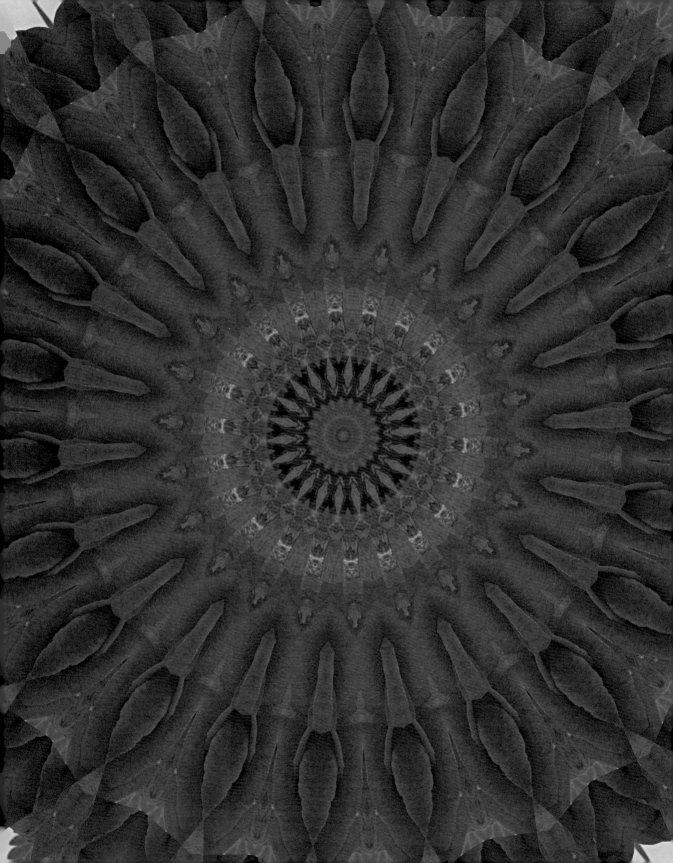

CHAPTER THREE

CRAFTING YOUR FIRST EXPERIENCE: THE CHEMISTRY OF PLEASURE

Learning to use cannabis for an enjoyable and safe experience every time is all about choices and boundaries. Almost everyone understands how to use alcohol appropriately, but very few of us were given an education about using cannabis appropriately due to prohibition and stigmas of the past. In this chapter, you will apply mindfulness and science to craft a cannabis experience—nonpsychoactive, euphoric, and any point in between that is right for you.

Mindfulness Exercise: Craft a First-Time Experience

"For this reason, we declare that pleasure is the beginning and end of a happy life. We are endowed by nature to recognize pleasure as the first and familiar good. Every choice and avoidance we make is guided by pleasure as our standard for judging the goodness of everything."[1]

Epicurus taught that moderation was the key to achieving the greatest pleasure and that overindulgence was the antithesis of his philosophy of pleasure as the greatest good. *Epicureanism* is the philosophy of the greatest good, pleasure, which Epicurus defined as a mind and body free of pain and anxiety. In this chapter, you will learn how to apply Epicurean principles of pleasure to your experiences with the cannabis plant.

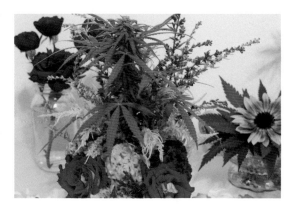

---

1   Epicurus, *Letter to Menoeceus*, Cook, Vincent Epicurus & Epicurean Philosophy https://epicurus.net/en /menoeceus.html

Most people experience a mix of curiosity and excitement when they try cannabis for the first time, whether that is a nonpsychoactive or euphoric experience. But I wouldn't be honest if I didn't tell you that sometimes, when people try cannabis for the first time, they may also experience fear or anxiety. If you are experiencing doubts, feelings of anxiety, or fear before trying psychotropic phytocannabinoids like THC for the first time, don't try these euphoria-inducing phytocannabinoids as a first-time cannabis experience. Instead, your "first time" should be a nonpsychoactive experience like a lotion, green vegetable, or CBD gummy.

For some, nonpsychoactive experiences with cannabis will be their favorite way to enjoy this plant the first time—and every time.

The effects of psychoactive phytocannabinoids like THC and THCV can't be compared to alcohol. Unlike alcohol, it's impossible to "overdose" in the classical sense. However, it is possible to create a very uncomfortable experience that may leave you in a psychologically vulnerable state of mind—and that can lead to physical responses like panic attacks or worse. As we have seen in previous chapters, oral consumption of phytocannabinoids in edibles is the most frequent cause of emergency room visits related to the over consumption of THC[2] due to the conversion of delta-9 THC to 11 Hydroxy THC in the liver—a more intense, potentially psychedelic, and longer lasting THC experience.[3] The good news is that you can avoid these experiences by preparing serving sizes of THC correctly.

Everyone wants to have a great experience with cannabis! A little planning goes a long way. Popping gummies or eating a brownie and expecting it to be like alcohol or prescription medication is unrealistic because cannabis is neither of these things. Think about the kind of experience you would like to have. Ideally, your answers to the following questions will reveal the kind of experience you want to have and the experience that is best suited for your personal needs and temperament.

1. **Do you want an euphoric experience?** If the answer is yes, move to question #2. If the answer is no, select the cannabinoids and/or plant products from chapter 2, and the recipes in this book that are nonpsychoactive, and write down some of those experiences

---

2 McCrimmon, Katie Kerwin. "Marijuana-related ER visits rising dramatically, edibles sparking particular concerns." UCHealth.org. https://www.uchealth.org/today/marijuana-related-er-visits-rising-dramatically-edibles-spraking-particular-concerns/

3 "11-Hydroxy-THC." Wikipedia https://en.wikipedia.org/wiki/11-Hydroxy-THC

that interest you the most. Next step: Try your hand at making some of these recipes and trying some of these nonpsychoactive experiences.

2. **Review the cannabinoid chemistry section of chapter 2 carefully, as you will be choosing the form of THC that you want to try.** You will be choosing between delta-9 THC / THCV (vaporized or smoked) and 11 Hydroxy THC (edibles). Write down what kind of experience you would like to have and any details such as where you would like to do this, and who you would like a psychoactive experience with cannabis in the beginning. I always recommend first time experiences with a friend.

   My first choice for a first-time THC cannabis experience will always be vaporized cannabis flower (delta-9 THC). The dose from vaporization is easy on the lungs because there is no smoke, it is easy to titrate exactly the dose and the length of the effects, and you will be immersed right away into the entourage chemistry of cannabis and aspects of tasting cannabis like you would wine or tea. It's also much more forgiving as the psychoactive effects only last about 2 to 4 hours.

3. **Consider how you may want to modify your euphoric experience—this can be done by pairing other cannabinoids and aromatics (terpenes) with THC.** A first experience may be the most enjoyable and provide the most relief if THC is paired 1:1 or greater CBD, for example.

4. **What are some of your favorite aromatics?** Do you enjoy the invigoration of citrus, the dreaminess of chamomile and cloves, or the relaxing scent of mint? Aromatherapy is a very effective enhancement for euphoric cannabis experiences. Fill a potpourri cooker with herbs or use an essential oil diffuser to enhance your experience. Enfleurage of cannabis flowers or resins will also create an aromatherapy experience.

5. **What are some of your favorite snacks?** You'll want to have plenty of your favorite snacks around or prepare a special meal the first time you try the psychoactive cannabinoid THC. Not only do they make the experience more enjoyable, but snacks or meals can also moderate the experience. Make a menu or a list of food and nonalcoholic beverages you would like to serve with your first euphoric cannabis experience.

6. **Write down some of your thoughts about using cannabis and why you have decided you would like to try cannabis. Are you seeking relief from pain or another symptom? Would you like to sleep better? Do you have anxiety? Would you just like to experience cannabis euphoria for leisure purposes like you would a glass of wine or**

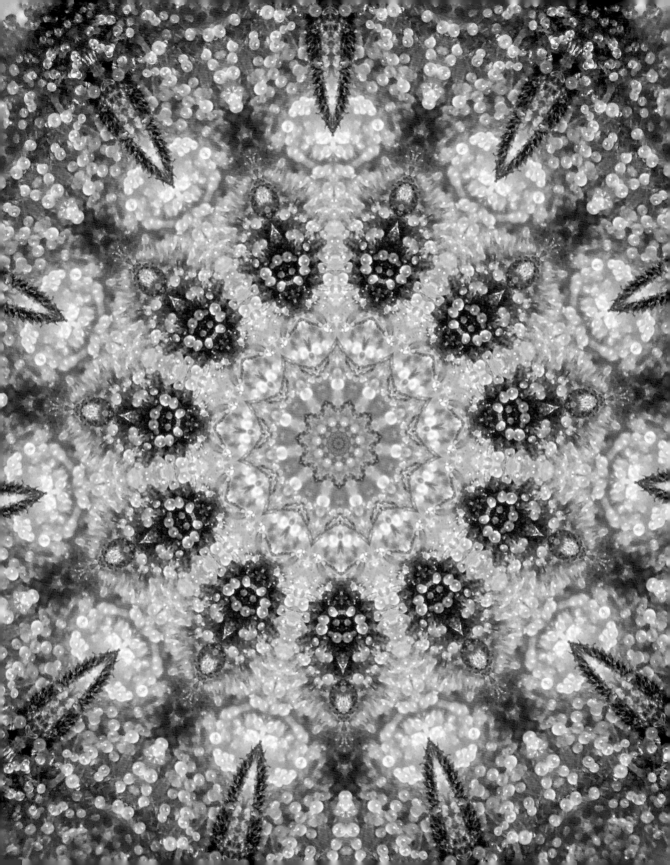

a cocktail? All of these answers are important because they will be a guide in terms of strain selection and the cannabinoid and aromatic (terpene) entourage you may want to pair with your THC experience.

What Does it Mean to "Get High"?

Generally speaking, what we mean by "getting high" is that we have consumed specifically delta-9 THC in a large enough dose to bring about the physiological and psychological changes associated with a variety of effects and feelings that are not part of our normal day-to-day bodily experiences. Your senses are altered, your mood changes, your thinking changes, your memory may be temporarily impaired, your reaction times slower, you may feel more euphoric or you may feel dysphoric based on the dose you have taken. The cannabis high is not like an alcohol high, yet both a share dose-dependent experience. Moderate use of alcohol can make one feel more sociable and somewhat euphoric in most cases. Moderate use of cannabis bears some similarity but with the added effects of unique sensory experiences that take center stage. The advantage of cannabis over alcohol is that cannabis has been shown to be safer than alcohol for your internal organs—and cannabis will never give you a hangover.[4]

Humans and animals like to "get high"—it's baked into our biology. Animals make use of the plants and other animals in their environment for psychoactive experiences.[5] My personal belief that the act of altering our senses and moods is perfectly healthy and natural in moderation is no doubt in conflict with the unwavering opinions of professional prohibitionists. However, I think that the opposition to our needs and natural tendencies, which are not so unlike the other creatures on this planet, is based more in puritanical control and shame than falsifiable evidence that "getting high" is always or even mostly harmful.

---

4 Lachenmeier, D. W., and J. Rehm. "Comparative risk assessment of alcohol, tobacco, cannabis and other illicit drugs using the margin of exposure approach." *Sci Rep*. 2015 Jan 30;5:8126. doi: 10.1038/srep08126. PMID: 25634572; PMCID: PMC4311234.
5 Arnold, Carrie. "No, Coyotes Don't Get High—But These Animals Do," *National Geographic Magazine* https://www.nationalgeographic.com/animals/article/160224-coyotes-mushrooms-drugs-high-animals-science

The Cardinal Rule of Your First Cannabis Experience: Start Low and Go Slow

Getting "high" off cannabis requires some effort. The phytocannabinoids THCA and THCVA from raw and cured cannabis flowers must be prepared correctly to have psychoactive effects. This is typically done with heat, which will instantly decarboxylate these cannabinoids. Smoking a joint or pipe will do this. Vaporizing cannabis flowers and concentrates in a heated vaporizer that produces no smoke will also decarboxylate these cannabinoids. Cooking the cannabinoids in edible substances, such as candy or brownies, or in oils, such as olive or coconut, will work too. Leaving cannabis in a hot car for a month or two will also result in decarboxylation—ikely unwanted decarboxylation, so don't do this one!

What dose of cannabinoids should I start with? This is the most common question a novice asks. If you are a medical cannabis patient, you have a medical cannabis card, or a recommendation from a doctor, the doctor will be your best resource for recommended starting doses and regular recommended doses.

As a general rule of thumb, a first-time oral dose of THC that will be tolerable and enjoyable will be anywhere from 1 to 5 milligrams. This dose may be fortified with other cannabinoids, as well, which will influence the effects of THC and enhance the benefits and positive effects. The most common cannabinoid to pair with THC is CBD, and you will see many products in the dispensary that have THC and CBD blended together. I like this blend.

While 1 to 5 milligrams is my suggested oral THC dose for a first-timer, it's actually my favorite dose as a long-timer, as well! After many years of writing cannabis books and using the cannabis plant, my I am particularly fond of edible THC (11 Hydroxy THC experience), with a dose range of 1 to 5 milligrams. I top out at 5 milligrams usually. There have been times I have taken 10 milligrams orally, but unless it is paired with twice as much CBD as THC, I don't really enjoy it as much as 5-milligram doses. I top out on pain relief at 10 milligrams THC. Anything more than 10 milligrams doesn't do anything additional to relieve chronic pain for me. Your experience may be different from mine, but until you have more experience with cannabis, starting low and going slow until you are very familiar with your tolerance levels will produce the most enjoyable experiences.

Essentially, 1 to 5 milligrams THC is the kind of oral dose that, if you happen to grow uncomfortable with it, won't last as long as if you took 50 milligrams THC. I've taken as much as 100 milligrams of THC in one setting as an edible, and it was not a fun day. Because

I was experienced and knew what was going on, I was able to control my anxiety, knowing that the psychoactive effects would abate within a few hours. I also used some of the remedies I describe later in this chapter to lessen the anxiety, and that worked very well for me.

Here is the summary of my suggestions for THC dosing for a beginner:

1. First choice will always be the delta-9 THC experience. Try this by using ground, cured cannabis flower in a vaporizer and inhaling the vapor 1 to 3 times. Wait 15 minutes, and if you would like more, inhale another 1 to 3 times.
2. Second choice is an edible tincture or candy (11 Hydroxy THC experience) with 1 to 5 milligrams of THC paired with the addition of CBD at the same amount or higher. Four milligrams THC and 8 milligrams of CBD is one of my favorite doses.
3. You could mix and match from these two. One inhale of vaporized cannabis flower and a gummy or mint with 2 milligrams THC and 8 milligrams CBD, or a blend of higher dose of CBD with no or little THC.
4. **Always wait 2 hours after you have taken THC orally before you take any additional oral doses**. Always wait at least 15 minutes after the first vaping or smoking session before vaping or smoking more.

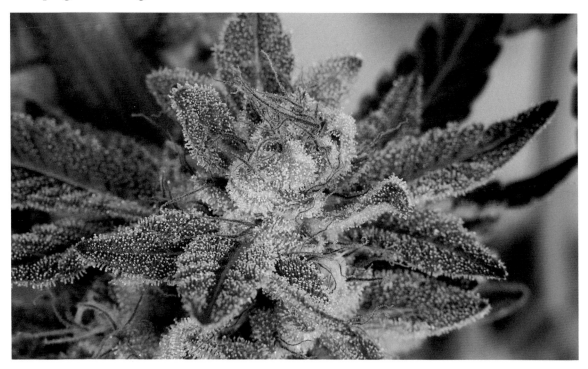

Fragrance and Tasting Lab: Learn to Taste Like the Connoisseurs Do!

Now that you know so much more about the chemistry of cannabis and the array of fragrance and flavors it can produce, you'll probably want to experience the finer aspects of learning to "taste" cannabis, just like you would wine, chocolate, or coffee!

Tasting is best done using a tabletop vaporizer or other good-quality raw plant material vaporizer that will not combust the plant material but will apply just enough heat to vaporize the phytocannabinoids and terpenes in the plant material. The full range of flavor can be tasted and evaluated when you do this. You may also taste concentrates and hashish with these vaporizers, as well.

If you'd like to do some tasting sessions, select several kinds of flower and grind each kind separately. On the side, you may have a small dish of coffee beans to sniff between each tasting. Some sparkling water that is plain or with a little lemon juice is also suggested for sipping. The coffee beans will clear your palate between tastings, and the sparkling water will refresh you.

Some people like to keep a tasting journal! This is a great way to review the flavors and the experiences that you have with different kinds of cannabis. When I got my first medical cannabis card two decades ago, I did tastings on a frequent basis to familiarize myself with the flavors and experiences that different kinds of cannabis have to offer. I would purchase 1 gram (which is plenty for tasting multiple times) of different kinds of flower and traditionally prepared hashish and do tastings with a friend. In this way, I discovered not only the flavors and chemistry profile that I enjoyed the most, but more importantly, the ones that were most effective for my chronic pain.

Managing Your Stash: Best Sanitary and Storage Practices with Cannabis

In this day and age, good sanitation practices are not only best practice, but they are essential for everyone's health and well-being. Based on this, there are some sanitary practice recommendations for consuming cannabis alone or with friends.

The primary best practice of cannabis storage is to store cannabis in a way that it does not develop any fungal contamination. This happens when cannabis is stored in a closed jar that has more than about 50 percent humidity. Sometimes, cannabis flowers can seem bone dry, and then after they are stored in a closed jar for a week, all of a sudden they have absorbed a lot of moisture and may even begin to take on a musty odor. If you detect a musty odor, the telltale sign of mold, you will need to dispose of these cannabis flowers.

Fortunately, prevention of fungal contamination is easy. You can purchase moisture absorption packets designed for use with cannabis flowers, or you can simply open your jar every couple of days to check for moisture. If there is too much humidity in the jar, leave the jar open for a day or two, shaking the jar to expose all of the plant material to dry air. Most people are opening their cannabis jars frequently enough that this kind of humidity problem is usually not a problem. But, if you find that you are only opening your storage jar once a week or so, you may want to check the contents a bit more frequently or use a moisture absorption pack.

Since you are already keeping your cannabis in a clean, dark, sealed jar, you probably have a few other accessories like a service tray and serving implements. Clean these frequently with 80 percent isopropyl or higher-proof alcohol. This is necessary due to the resins left behind when preparing cannabis flowers and concentrates. Keep all mouthpieces and other implements that come in contact with your mouth clean with the same strength of alcohol.

Make a Fruit Pipe for Single-Person Service

Instead of sharing vapor mouthpieces, joints, and glassware service at parties and gatherings, cut fruit like citrus or even apples into smoking implements for each guest. This is a very tasty and attractive way to serve guests, as the fruit adds additional flavor and terpene content to the smoking experience.

Materials

Large oranges, lemons, or grapefruits
Small carving knife
Poking implement (ice pick or skewer)

Directions

1. First, you will need to carve a little bowl shape on the top end of the fruit, and then use your poking implement to poke through the middle of the carved bowl area to the opposite end of the fruit, creating a tunnel.

2. Pull out the poker and push it through the tunnel to the exit hole you just created on the opposite side (this is where you will put your mouth to inhale), and use the poker to enlarge the tunnel from the exit hole to the bowl on top enough so that air can be drawn through when using the exit hole as a mouthpiece.

3. Cannabis flower or hashish will be loaded into the bowl on the top and lit. Smoke will be inhaled through the exit hole. At the end of the gathering or party, all of the fruit can be collected and added to the compost pile or thrown away.

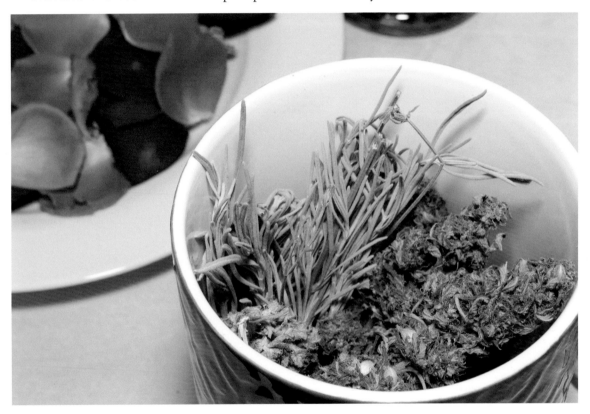

Recipe: Cannabis Flower Enfleurage

Enfleurage is a kind of French perfumery technique dating back hundreds of years. It involves transferring the terpenes of delicate herbs or flowers directly to a solid fat. You do this by first spreading the solid fat across a glass plate and then placing the flowers and herbs on top of this. Leave it for a day or a few days, remove the herbs or flowers, and then repeat the process several times with another batch of fresh aromatics spread out on the same glass plate with the fat until the fat is infused with copious amounts of terpenes from the aromatic plant material.

The same kind of enfleurage technique can be done in different ways and is not limited to solid fats. You can use the resins of cannabis in order to infuse them with various terpene profiles. The simplest method that has been in practice for more years than I can count was the simple act of storing dried, cured cannabis flowers with dried orange peels. In prohibition years, this practice was often employed for the less-than-stellar "brick weed," which was often tasteless.

If you would like to enfleurage your cannabis flowers, the recipe is quite simple:

Materials
Dried aromatic plants (your preference)
Cannabis flowers
Dark glass jar (amber or Miron glass) with tight-fitting lid

Directions
1. Select any dried aromatic plants that you prefer. This can be anything, like dried orange peels, dried lavender, dried rosemary, white peppercorns, dried rose petals, dried mint leaves, etc. The main rule of thumb on this is that your aromatic plant material must be fresh and fragrant but very dry.
2. You will need a dark glass jar (amber or Miron glass is preferred) with a tight-fitting lid. Layer your cannabis flowers with the aromatic plant material in a separate layer so that the aromatics are easy to remove when the process is complete.
3. Close the jar for 2 days. After this, open the jar and check that the contents of the jar do not seem moist in any way. If it does, leave the jar open for a day or two and shift the contents a bit until the material is very dry again. Close the jar again for 2 to 3 days. When you open it again, everything should be just about as dry as when you closed the jar. If it is not, open the jar and shift the contents again to expose it to the air.
4. After about a week, the aromatics will impart their fragrances to the cannabis flowers. You may taste these as is, or you may want to do another round of enfleurage with more dried aromatic material.
5. When the cannabis flowers are infused to your satisfaction, remove the aromatic plant material and store the cannabis flowers in the tightly closed jar. Enjoy!

Rules of the Road: Stay Safe, Know Your Limits, Prepare Ahead

If you are reading this book, you're already an adult eighteen or over who understands the gravity of driving, or performing any other critical task requiring clear thinking and sharp motor skills, while under the influence of cannabinoids. Mindfully consider what you will need to do for the rest of the day or evening before you use cannabis. Make note of what experience you have chosen (the shorter acting experience of delta-9 THC, or the longer acting and more intense experience of 11 Hydroxy THC) and plan your session with cannabis accordingly. And when in doubt, stay home or call a car service or your designated driver.

Most people who are experienced with using cannabis have had at least one uncomfortable experience. These are rare, but they can happen. If you've used cannabis and you feel uncomfortable, there are two things you can do that will lessen the discomfort:

The first one has been described in many medical texts from the nineteenth century when the patient's experience with a cannabis dose they were given becomes uncomfortable: lemon juice. Lemon juice is an excellent remedy if you feel that you've had a little too much cannabis, or you do not like the way that you feel. Preparing a delicious glass or pitcher of lemonade using real lemon juice is not only helpful for the inevitable dry mouth that is very common with THC, but it is also helpful in regulating the THC high.

The second one, which as far as I can determine was the invention of rocker Neil Young, is to prepare a closed jar of fresh peppercorns (not ground pepper, which will make you sneeze) and inhale the aroma of the peppercorns and/or chew a peppercorn from the jar if you feel any anxiety after you have used cannabis. Many people, including myself, have successfully used this method to alleviate the rare instances when you've had just a little too much cannabis or you feel uncomfortable or anxious. We theorize that this works because peppercorns contain a terpene, beta-caryophyllene, very similar to cannabinoids and it attaches itself to cannabinoid receptors. I haven't been able to find any studies on this, but it's a very tried-and-true method of relieving discomfort from a dose of cannabinoids in the cannabis community.

Another method to try is combining these two ingredients in a warm beverage. Warm some fresh lemonade and a few peppercorns in a cup in the microwave or a pan on the stove and enjoy. This is the one I like if I've overindulged with an edible THC product. Sipping on the hot peppercorn lemonade is as delicious as it is helpful.

Finally, one of the most reliable methods of lessening the effects of THC is to eat something. Eating a nutritious meal high in fat is quite effective from anecdotal experience. Cheese, fruit, and crackers is an ideal fast meal idea in this scenario. Don't forget to have some hot lemon and peppercorn tea or lemonade on the side.

Keep in mind that none of these methods are appropriate to use in order to drive a car or use dangerous machinery while under the influence of THC. Only time can deliver the complete baseline functioning necessary to do these things. **These home remedies are not a substitute for the clear thinking and sharp motor skills required to drive or do other critical activities.**

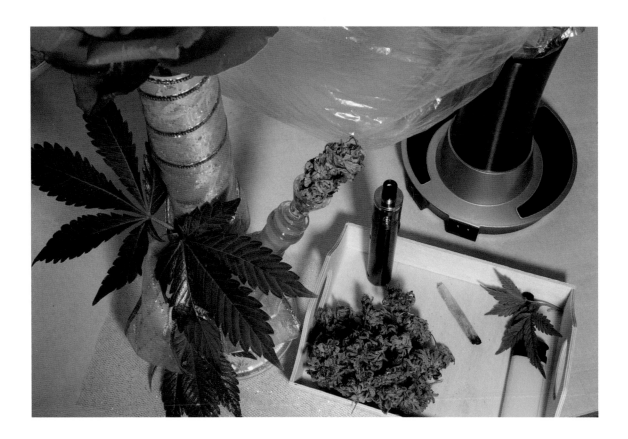

Vaporizing or Smoking or Edibles?

Smoking anything has lost its appeal for many in the twenty-first century. And for good reasons: inhaling combusted plant material is not healthy practice. Doctors who write medical cannabis recommendations often advise patients to use a vaporizer instead of smoking, especially if you have conditions already compromising your health.

Using a clean pipe or even smoking a joint occasionally, in my experience, has not compromised my health, and I know of many others who indulge this way on occasion, as well. But it certainly is an issue for your personal doctor, or the doctor who has written your medical cannabis recommendation, to advise on what will be best for you.

Edibles have often been the first choice of cannabis novices. If this is going to be your first choice, and you want to ensure that your 11 Hydroxy THC experience is a good experience, it's best to purchase premeasured and tested edibles from a legal dispensary, such as gummy bears, as opposed to making an edible at home for your first time. 11 Hydroxy THC in small doses can have very powerful pain and inflammation relief effects—a small dose will go a long way during your first and subsequent experiences as a cannabis novice. Only purchase edible products with single-serving doses of 1 to 5 milligrams of THC for your first experiences until you are sure of your tolerance levels. I discourage beginners from purchasing single-serving products with a large amount of THC (25, 50, or 100 milligrams) and attempting to split these into usable doses. If you forget the doses or confuse the product with something else, you could be in for a very uncomfortable experience, so stick with the premeasured, 1- to 5-milligram single-serving doses typically found in products like gummies or jellies.

Remember, Cannabis Is Not for Everyone

How wonderful it would be if everyone could enjoy and benefit from every plant in the world! Realistically, we know that's not possible. For those of us who love cannabis as much as we love many other beneficial herbs, we want everyone to enjoy cannabis as much as we do as a medicinal, spiritual, and euphoric plant! But it is not possible to predict who will enjoy or benefit from cannabis. **This is yet one more reason why it is always suggested that new users of euphoric cannabis products start low and go slow—the cardinal rule of first-time cannabis consumption!**

Let's dive into the reasons why cannabis is not for everyone:

- **Mental Illness:** There's a long-standing debate in the scientific and medical community about the effects of cannabis on mental illness. Some of this debate appears to be reasonable, while some of it sounds like a repeat of "Reefer Madness." The best evidence right now tells us that cannabis (in particular, THC) doesn't cause schizophrenia; someone has to already have the genetic predisposition for schizophrenia to develop this mental illness. If THC-rich cannabis causes mental illness, we should see an uptick in schizophrenia cases, especially in the US states where cannabis has been legal for more than a decade. We do not see a rise in schizophrenia diagnosis to correlate with a rise in cannabis legalization.[6] For someone who has a mental illness or a history of addiction, or has previously been diagnosed

---

6 Carey, Benedict, "Does Marijuana Use Cause Schizophrenia?" *New York Times*, January 2019 https://www.nytimes.com/2019/01/17/health/cannabis-marijuana-schizophrenia.html

with a mental illness, a consultation with a licensed physician who is knowledgeable about cannabis is an important first step before using or continuing to use cannabis products of any kind.

- **Medical Contraindication:** You may be taking a medication or therapy that is not compatible with cannabis. Always speak to a licensed physician about your specific health needs and cannabis use.
- **Cannabis Hyperemesis Syndrome:** This is a well-documented condition, typically in people who have been using cannabis in high doses for extended periods of time. It is a rare but very real condition. Most heavy users of cannabis will never develop this condition, but for those who do, **the only cure is complete cessation of all cannabis intake forever**. CHS causes frequent vomiting that can lead to dehydration or dangerous electrolyte imbalance. If you begin vomiting after using cannabis, take a long, hot shower (hot showers appear to relieve the symptoms quickly), stop using cannabis immediately, and seek advice from a licensed physician knowledgeable about cannabis and CHS.[7] Doctors cannot predict who will develop this rare condition, and for many frequent and high-dose consumers, it never happens. Because this rare condition generally develops in people who consume cannabis frequently and in larger doses, and not in moderate users of cannabis, perhaps one of the best ways to always ensure that you will be able to enjoy cannabis in the future is to always consume in moderation.
- **Cannabis Allergy:** This is another contraindication for the continued use of cannabis if the allergic reaction is due to the cannabis itself. There are several possibilities if one has an allergic reaction to cannabis:
  1. The cannabis has mold or yeasts growing on it or is contaminated with pesticides or another chemical, and the allergic reaction is to one or more of these things. Never use any part of the cannabis plant, including flowers, that has a musty or "dirty" odor or shows signs of decomposition. This is not a cannabis allergy; it is an allergy to another organism growing with or on the cannabis, and reactions to this cannabis will resolve if clean cannabis is consumed.

---

7 "Cannabis Hypermeisis Syndrome Fact Sheet," Cedars Sinai https://www.cedars-sinai.org/health-library/diseases-and-conditions/c/cannabinoid-hyperemesis-syndrome.html

2. The allergic reaction may be to cannabis pollen. Only male and hermaphrodite plants produce pollen, so this should not be an issue if one is exposed only to the female plants. It can be an issue for people with cannabis pollen allergies who live in rural areas with hemp farming.[8]

3. The allergic reaction is to any part of the cannabis plant, including the terpenes, male, female, or hermaphrodite plants.

4. The allergic reaction is a food allergy to cannabis seeds or other nonpsychoactive parts of the cannabis plant. According to the American Academy of Allergy, Asthma & Immunology, cannabis allergy is cross-reactive with other foods with similar proteins that occur in cannabis: "In addition there is reported cross-reactivity between marijuana and certain foods. Cannabis cross-reacting foods that have been reported to cause allergy include tomato, peach and hazelnut. This is due to cross-reacting proteins or allergens found both in marijuana and these foods. This cross-reactivity can potentially cause serious allergic reactions. The important and relevant allergens still require research and clinical definition."[9]

- **You don't like cannabis, or any nonspecific symptom or preference**. Cannabis is not for everyone, and if you find that you do not like cannabis, you are under no obligation to explain why. No one has ever asked me to explain why I don't like valerian (because it smells like dirty socks); there's nothing wrong with valerian, I just don't like the smell. No one has ever pressured me into using valerian or cannabis. Etiquette around cannabis and plant medicine culture as a whole is such that if you find you do not like cannabis, it's very likely that no one will ever pressure you to use it. So relax.

---

8 Mayoral, M., H. Calderón, R. Cano, and M. Lombardero. "Allergic rhinoconjunctivitis caused by Cannabis sativa pollen." *J Investig Allergol Clin Immunol.* 2008; 18(1):73-4. PMID: 18361109. http://www.jiaci.org/issues/vol18issue1/13-17.pdf

9 "Marijuana Cannabis Allergy." *American Academy of Allergy, Asthma & Immunology* https://www.aaaai.org/tools-for-the-public/conditions-library/allergies/marijuana-cannabis-allergy#:~:text=Breathing%20or%20inhaling%20marijuana%20allergens,Anaphylaxis%20has%20also%20been%20reported.

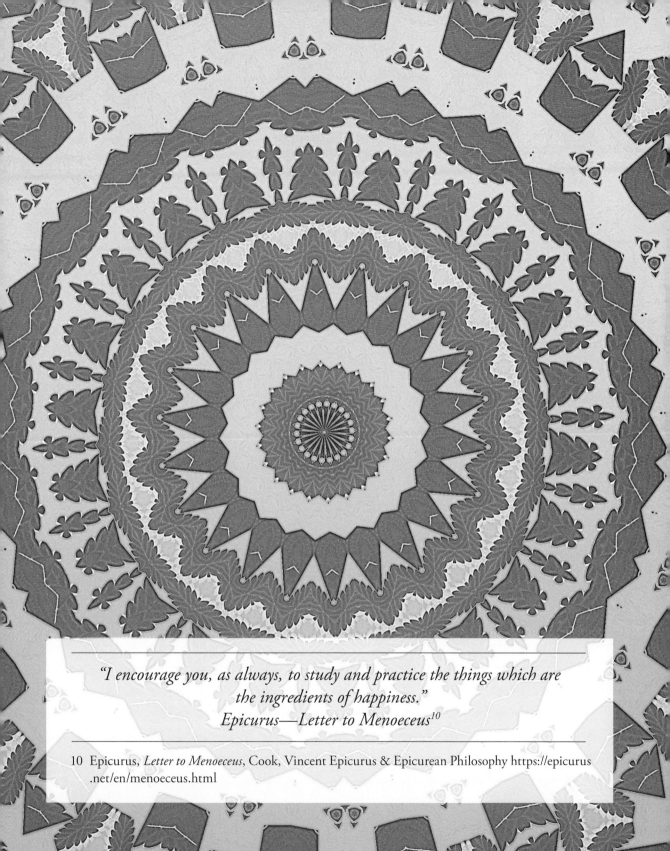

"I encourage you, as always, to study and practice the things which are
the ingredients of happiness."
Epicurus—Letter to Menoeceus[10]

10 Epicurus, *Letter to Menoeceus*, Cook, Vincent Epicurus & Epicurean Philosophy https://epicurus
.net/en/menoeceus.html

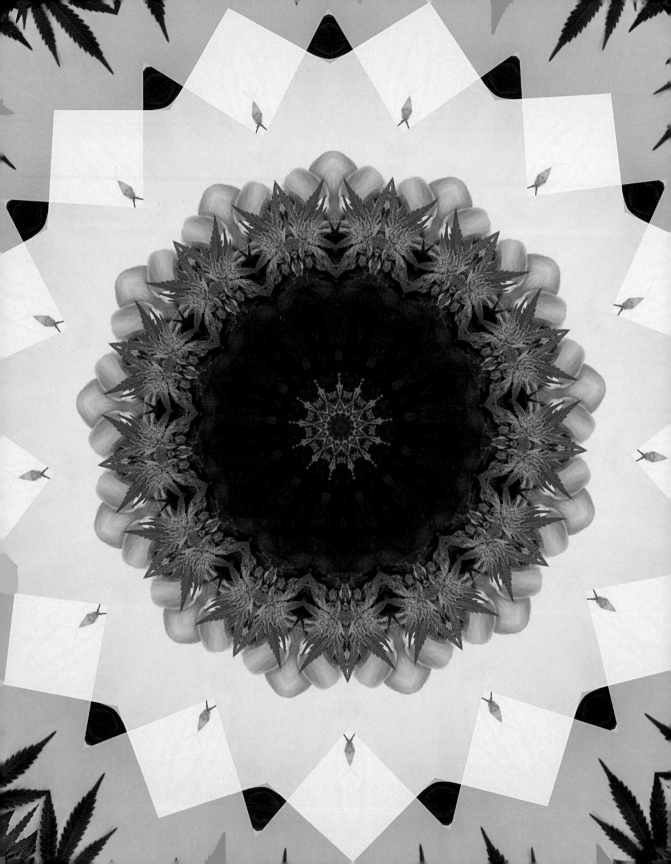

CHAPTER FOUR

LET'S GO SHOPPING! GET READY FOR YOUR FIRST LEGAL CANNABIS DISPENSARY VISIT

Navigating a legal cannabis dispensary for the first time can be very challenging for a beginner. In this chapter, you will find out why that is and how to have a satisfying trip to the cannabis dispensary of your choice. Not all dispensaries are alike; and as of the publication date of this book, there is very little regulation as to how the staff of a dispensary can serve you and what they can tell you apart from the labeled testing requirements for every product they carry as specified by your local laws and regulations. Learn to be your own "budtender" and take control of your dispensary experience!

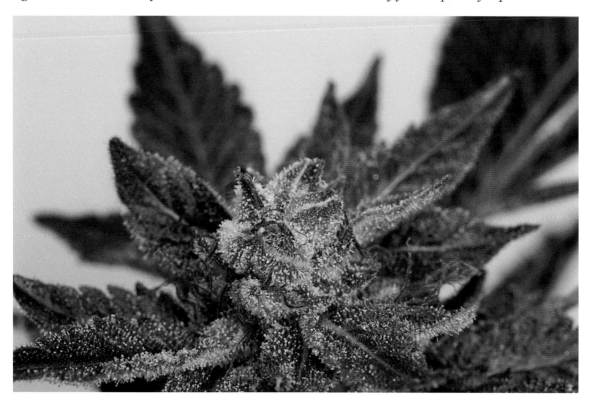

Medical or Leisure? Understanding the Differences

In most states where cannabis is legal, the difference between a medical or leisure dispensary isn't apparent in the products offered. The products offered in either kind of dispensary will be the same. Some states have only medical dispensaries, and to shop at these dispensaries, you will need to meet the legal requirements of your state, which will typically involve visiting with a licensed physician and receiving a written recommendation.

In Oregon, our dispensaries serve both medical and leisure. The products are the same. The difference between the two is that prices at the dispensary are slightly lower for medical cardholders, and the law allows you to grow more plants in your home. Even though I personally use cannabis for medicinal purposes, I don't bother getting a medical card here, because they cost $200 and the discount at the dispensary isn't that much. Also, I can only grow six plants as a medical cardholder. For simple adult leisure grows, the law allows for four plants of any size. This number of plants is sufficient for my medicinal needs.

Before you visit a dispensary for the first time, you will need to ascertain what the requirements are in your state and be able to meet those requirements. For example, here in Oregon, all I need to do is show a driver's license. But, in medical states, you will need to show your ID and your medical card or recommendation from your physician to the person hosting the counter upon entry at the dispensary.

If you are a senior citizen or disabled, and you are in a legal cannabis state, some companies offer buses for free transportation to and from the dispensaries. If you are interested in visiting a few dispensaries at a time, check around and see if there are any services offering dispensary tours for seniors. This has become somewhat commonplace in some medical cannabis states.

Selecting and Evaluating Dispensaries

The most important thing when selecting a dispensary to visit nowadays is cleanliness. Not all dispensaries operate with the kinds of principles in regards to sanitary practices that we've all become accustomed to in this day and age. Checking Google reviews online is a very good way to see what others are saying about the condition of the store, the staff, the selection, and the pricing.

Why is cleanliness so important? Because cleanliness reflects the care that the ownership of the store takes when selecting products, employees, and services that are all part of the business. Owners that care about the health and safety of the customer are going to provide an overall better customer experience. Small mom-and-pop dispensaries can be as fresh and clean as a larger chain store; size doesn't matter as much as the customer experience matters.

Some dispensaries are more expensive to shop in than other dispensaries. These higher-end dispensaries may or may not be offering products in line with the prices they are charging. It's not cheap to grow superb indoor cannabis flowers. Most of the "top shelf" offerings available at dispensaries will be the kind of flowers that have wow factor in terms of color, fragrance, and phytocannabinoid content. Prices need to be in line with what is being offered for sale. For example, the sun-grown flower, which happens to be my favorite, is not as pricey or exceptionally gorgeous as many indoor grown flowers, but it has the "salt of the earth" appeal and will have more variety in terms of plant chemistry.

Overall, a good dispensary will have product offerings at all price points, and all of these products should be of good quality. Just because you're paying less for something doesn't mean quality has to suffer.

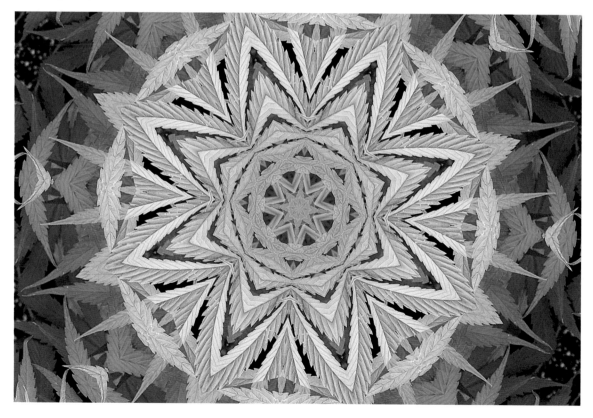

Commercial Products Sold in Dispensaries

The first thing I always hear from those who are new to the cannabis dispensary experience is how the experience made them feel like a kid in a candy store and how they ended up dropping three hundred dollars on their first visit. I still remember my first legal dispensary visit back in 2006 and how I dropped three hundred dollars! If you have it to spend, knock yourself out! The "candy store" feeling is quite apropos, as these establishments almost always have so much to choose from. There may be thirty or more choices of cured flowers, as many concentrates, fifty kinds of edibles, and an entire suite of spa products. Alternatively, smaller mom-and-pop dispensaries may only have five or ten kinds of flowers, a half-dozen concentrates, and as many edible products along with a lotion or two. These smaller shops are also worth your time to explore because quite often, as a mom-and-pop establishment, they may be closely tied to craft farmers who grow or manufacture unique products.

Some of the kinds of products you will encounter in a dispensary include:

Cured Whole Flowers

These are sold in amounts as little as 1 gram. Most whole plant products like flower and even concentrates will be sold in metric units of grams. They will typically be classed into:

Top-shelf: The most expensive flower in the shop with high sensory appeal, such as a unique color and fragrance. Top shelf is almost always artisanally manicured by hand. It's indoor-grown cannabis with very high phytocannabinoid content or a unique indoor or outdoor flower with very specialized phytocannabinoid and terpene content. Indoor-grown, top-shelf cannabis is significantly more expensive to grow than outdoor-grown cannabis, and this is one of the factors that contributes to this cannabis product being sold for premium prices. Depending on who you ask, it's not necessarily the "best" cannabis flower for sale in the dispensary.

Mid-shelf: This is where most sun-grown cannabis will be placed in the shop. Sun-grown, otherwise known as outdoor grown, has more farm-to-table appeal, and it can provide some impressive sensory input on par with indoor grown cannabis. It's more earthy, reflecting the influences of its terroir. Craft farmers grow in pristine outdoor conditions, with influences of the special qualities of the land itself, sometimes known as terroir. This is a term often used in the wine industry regarding the location of a vineyard and the qualities it imparts to the wine. Indoor grown cannabis does not have terroir; its qualities are due to the artificial environment it is grown in. Sun-grown cannabis may be slightly lower in phytocannabinoid content than top-shelf with 15 to 20 percent phytocannabinoid content as opposed to top-shelf offerings, which can be as high as 28 percent in some cases. But that doesn't mean that top-shelf is "better" than mid-shelf or sun-grown! Sun-grown is also very environmentally friendly when grown by craft farmers who use sustainable methods of water and crop management.

"Bargain bud" or bottom-shelf: These cannabis flower products can be a mix of indoor and outdoor grown, "popcorn buds" (smaller buds further down on the stem of the cannabis plant), "trim" (sugar leaf trim from the harvest manicure), flowers that seeded a little bit, flowers close to the expiration date, or a just good deal the dispensary was able to obtain for a bulk order. You can find good deals on good cannabis flowers on the bottom shelf. The phytocannabinoid content will vary. I have seen drop-dead gorgeous CBD-rich cannabis flowers sold at a discount on the bottom shelf with 17 percent CBD (that's high for CBD content) but little or no THC. You may find indoor grown "popcorn buds" that came from the same cannabis plants that produced an indoor top-shelf flower, with a similar phytocannabinoid content as the top-shelf flower, but they are being sold for less for aesthetic reasons.

Tips for Evaluating Cured Cannabis Flowers

1. A dispensary should provide a hygienic way for the customer to experience the aroma of the flowers it has for sale. Typically, this will be "fragrance jars" with a few grams of the flower that can be sniffed. Some dispensaries will open the jar they are serving from and wave the fragrance from the jar so that you can smell it. I'm not fond of dispensaries that allow every customer to put their nose in the same gallon-sized jar they are dispensing from. But, if you are purchasing whole cannabis flower, it is customary for there to be a way for you to sample the fragrance before buying. This is important not just for aesthetic pleasure, but also gives you the opportunity to detect musty odors, cannabis that smells stale, or lack of any fragrance at all. Most dispensaries are

(Continued on next page)

---

required by their locale to test for the presence of mold before the products are put on the shelf. But after they have been on the shelf for a while, if the dispensary is not adept at managing their cured flower inventory, they could develop a "musty" odor, which is the tell-tale sign of mold.

2. You should be given a clear view of the flowers that you will be purchasing or be allowed to select from a jar which flowers you would like to purchase.

3. Many dispensaries provide table-top magnification lights that customers can use to view cannabis flowers up close. If this is not the case, you can obtain a very inexpensive magnification tool called a jeweler's loupe. This is a small magnification glass with at least 10X magnification. You can use this to view the trichomes on the flowers in order to determine the quality.

4. Check the harvest dates on the labels. The best cured flowers will be no more than six months from the date of harvest.

Concentrates and Hashish

Concentrated phytocannabinoid products: These are among the most popular products in any dispensary. They are often more convenient to use because they are concentrated. These products are popular with connoisseurs and people who are seasoned cannabis consumers. Beginners should be cautious using these products until they understand their tolerance for various phytocannabinoids.

Full-extract cannabis oil / RSO: This is a thick, concentrated cannabis oil produced by ethyl alcohol extraction. The alcohol is evaporated, and what remains is a blackish-green oil that almost resembles fresh tar due to the color imparted by the concentrated chlorophyll. This product should not be used for vaping or smoking because of the chlorophyll content. This product can be taken plain on the tongue (which may result in a 11 Hydroxy THC experience, beginners are urged to be cautious with using this product orally), or used in various edible or topical/transdermal products. This product is quite popular with medical cannabis card holders for various medicinal applications as well.

Live rosin: This concentrated product represent the top-shelf, the most expensive concentrate products carried in dispensaries. This is a rarified product and are made by applying a small amount of heat to cannabis flower and/or pressing it under very high pressure to literally squeeze the resins out of the cannabis flower. They are rich in terpene content as well as phytocannabinoid content. Some of the most impressive ones I've experienced have the fragrance of a bag of oranges or true vanilla custard. The terpenes are just that powerful in these live rosin concentrated products. They are used in vape pens, vaporizers, and in glass service for "dabs." They are among the highest in phytocannabinoid content of all concentrate products.

CO_2: When extraction of cannabis resins is completed by using carbon dioxide. This is a clean, petroleum-free method of producing a concentrated product that can be used in vaporizers or glass service. CO_2 extractions, live resin or rosin, will not contain any plant material and will be pure.

Traditional hashish formulations / temple balls / hand-rolled: When a dispensary carries these products, produced by the masters of the craft, it is indeed a special dispensary. These concentrate products may be slightly lower in phytocannabinoid content than resins or the more pure extractions of phytocannabinoids because they will almost always contain some plant material due to the rustic methods of production. These methods date back thousands of years. They are hand-rolled and manipulated in precise ways to create an end product that will reflect the terroir of the cannabis flower (and outdoor or sun-grown cannabis is preferred for making these kinds of hashish) and contain all of the entourage of the flower such as the terpenes. Some of these hashishes are aged and also develop new terpenes and entourage during that process. Like other concentrated products, caution is urged for beginners. However, I would recommend these traditional hashish formulas for beginners who want to try a concentrated product for the first time.

Cold water hashish / ice water hashish / bubble hash: These are another kind of hashish produced by sieving the trichomes away from most of the green plant material using cold water and/or ice to freeze the plant material. It's a clean method that makes a pretty good product. In my experience, it tends to be a less intensive terpene experience. These concentrates retain a small amount of plant material that will make them lower in total phytocannabinoids. They are, generally speaking, among the lower-priced concentrate products available in the dispensary. They are a convenient and inexpensive way to buy measured amounts of phytocannabinoids for various recipes.

Kif / pressed cake / dry ice: Another clean and solventless method of producing concentrated phytocannabinoids. Depending on the method used to make these, either by shaking trichomes from plant material and pressing it into a small cake or by the use of dry ice (frozen CO_2), these products may be more similar to traditional hashish or similar to resin/ rosin/CO_2 products. Products made with dry ice are going to be higher in phytocannabinoid content and products made by shaking and sifting are going to be a little lower due to the small amount of plant material that remains in the product. In my experience, these products, if packaged correctly, can retain a lot of the terpenes that can make for quite a sensory experience.

Cannabis flower rolled with/coated in concentrated product: Sometimes these products are called moon rocks or moonstones—they are whole cannabis flowers that have been rolled with, dipped in, or coated with a concentrated cannabis product. This product is intended for smoking or vaporizing purposes only. The quality of these concentrated products will vary. If you are interested in trying these, try to ascertain the origin of all the plant material and the type of concentrate used to enrich the flowers before purchasing.

Solvent-extracted hashish oil / wax / shatter: These products have fallen out of favor for many. There is a good reason for this: these products are produced using petroleum distillate solvents. More than a decade ago, these were among the most common concentrates found in dispensaries. Apart from being dangerous to produce, environmentally hazardous, and generally speaking, a concentrate product that lacks in all of the aesthetic and entourage qualities of the other concentrated products here, they are much lower quality than a live rosin or even a traditional hashish product. Petroleum solvents simply ruin everything else the cannabis flower has to offer, except for the phytocannabinoids. Nowadays, these products are sold more cheaply than products like live rosin or CO_2 products. I would skip over these if you find them at a dispensary. Always confirm with dispensary staff that the product you are purchasing is not extracted with solvents if you want to avoid these products.

> ## Tips for Evaluating Concentrated Cannabis Products
>
> 1. Always read labels. Because the packaging of these products can be very small, designed for packaging 1 to 2 grams' worth of concentrated product, labels may be quite small. A magnifying glass or jeweler's loupe can aid in your effort to read and understand labeling. Look for the date of manufacture—only purchase concentrate products within the three-month window of manufacture.
> 2. The only exception to this rule would be some of the traditionally prepared hashish products, which are sometimes aged as part of the process.
> 3. Some concentrated products will be offered to the customer for fragrance sampling. Typically, this will be one small container set aside for this purpose as opposed to breaking the seal on fresh product. Take advantage of this offer when it is presented to you at the concentrates counter.

Prepared Smokeable and Vaping Products

Pre-rolls / joints: This is another common product offering you will find in your favorite dispensaries. The first thing you will notice about these products is that they are quite large and packaged using a method known as "cone-rolling" and will look similar to a cone shape. These products may or may not have concentrated products added to them, so it is advisable to carefully read all labeling on a pre-roll product. Although these are whole-flower products, you will not have the opportunity to sample the fragrance or view the original flower material they are made from. Out west, these are a favorite product for a day at the beach because they are convenient, and unlike tobacco cigarettes with poly fiber filters, pre-rolls are all organic material that readily degrades if they are dropped or snuffed out in the sand.

Vape scts and cartridges: There's a lot of buzz around vapor products these days. My personal opinion is that these are safe products to use if the company making them is reliable with the hardware they manufacture and if the oils used in the cartridges are produced without the use of petroleum solvents. Look for a product manufacturer with good reviews and a professional product. Cheap-looking vapes are going to be just that: cheap. Quality vape products are not cheap products, but these products are usually a good bang for the buck because they last for a long time. Most people find that inhaling one time from a vape is enough. Good cartridges can last for as long as fifty inhales.

Tips for Evaluating Prepared Smokeable and Vape Products

1. Check labeling carefully for manufacture dates and for the kind of oil product that is inside the cartridge. Cartridges need to be within three months of manufacture date, at minimum.

2. If you are also purchasing the hardware to use the cartridge from the dispensary, go online and check reviews and information about the company that has manufactured this hardware.

3. Cones/pre-rolls/joints also have harvest and/or manufacturing dates. Look for fresh products in this category and check that all seals are intact on the packaging. Don't buy loose pre-rolls that are not in protective packaging.

Edible Phytocannabinoid Products

These products will result in a 11 Hydroxy THC experience if the product has delta-9 THC in it. As we have learned in earlier chapters, the 11 Hydroxy THC experience is much more intense and longer lasting than the delta-9 THC that is experienced by vaping, smoking, mucous membrane penetration, or topical applications. Edible products with a mix of THC and CBD are highly recommended for beginners that want to try edible products for the first time.

Candy / lozenges: Gummies, hard candy, cough drops, and taffy, comprise most of the candy-type products you will find in a dispensary. As far as edible products go, these are usually more predictable for a beginner because each gummy or candy will have only a fraction of the total THC content of the entire package. Look for products that are **not** infused with petroleum solvent–extracted cannabis oil.

Bakery goods: The array of products included in this category includes any bakery item, cookies, brownies, cakes, and muffins. Single-serving packaged bakery products are edible products that beginners need to be especially mindful of due to the fact that they can contain very high amounts of phytocannabinoids and require a consumer to cut or portion them several ways to take a smaller dose. Always read labels carefully. Look for products that are **not** infused with petroleum solvent–extracted cannabis oil.

Confectionary: Chocolate, fudge, brittle, and truffle-like products comprise most of this category. These can be whole single candy bars or small bites. Be aware that products like candy bars may need to be portioned due to the high phytocannabinoid content. Always read the label. Look for products that are **not** infused with petroleum solvent–extracted cannabis oil.

Snacks and nuts: These products are usually packaged in small bags similar to mainstream single-serving products like potato chips. Like many other edible products, the entire single-serving packaged product can contain soaring amounts of phytocannabinoid and must be portioned by the consumer into smaller amounts. Always read the label to ascertain how many portions you will have to divide these products into in order to get a safe serving for yourself. Look for products that are **not** infused with petroleum solvent–extracted cannabis oil.

Prepared meal / pizza: This is a really fun (for some!) type of product you will find in a dispensary. I recall from a few years ago that a dispensary I used to frequent had frozen, cannabis-infused Thanksgiving dinners every holiday season that were about the size of a TV dinner. These also contained around 100 milligrams of THC, which means that this product isn't at all appropriate for a beginner. Ditto on frozen pizza slices. I haven't seen these products in the dispensaries I frequent nowadays, but I am sure they're still out there. Be cautious and aware that if you purchase these products (and I don't recommend them for beginners), you are going to have to cook and then portion and refrigerate in order to use them. Read all of the labeling very carefully. Look for products that are **not** infused with petroleum solvent–extracted cannabis oil.

Ice cream: Frozen confections will be packaged in small pint-sized containers. What's great about these is that they require no cooking, and you can eat a spoonful at a time. Read the label carefully to calculate how much phytocannabinoid will be in every spoonful you consume. Look for products that are **not** infused with petroleum solvent-extracted cannabis oil.

Gluten-free, allergen-free products: I urge caution with products claiming to be allergen-free or gluten-free that are sold in dispensaries at the time of writing this book. The same regulation required by law from mainstream food and beverage manufacturers does not always apply to products sold in cannabis dispensaries. As someone who carries EpiPens for life-threatening anaphylactic food allergies, I urge caution to others with similar medical issues. In many, but not all, cases, these products were created to meet customer demand for a trend in diet habits, not medical issues. I think this is going to change in the future to reflect the same standards of mainstream food manufacturing. With new US states and international locales legalizing cannabis every year, more competition and higher standards will shape these products in the future.

The problem is that it's hard to tell what products actually meet the criteria of "safe" for an allergic or celiac population. One of my personal experiences with this involved a product advertising itself directly to people with food allergies as being "free of allergens." A call to the company to receive clarification on the ingredients and production process of this product ended with the answer "that's proprietary." The company had made the decision not to serve an allergic patient by refusing to disclose ingredients and production processes while continuing to advertise as "free of allergens." **Only cannabis companies who make products with full disclosure could ever be considered safe for the allergic or celiac communities, just as companies who manufacture mainstream food products serving allergic and celiac populations do.**

Tips for Evaluating Edible Products

1. Read labels carefully to determine if portioning will be required and to check the manufacturing date. Don't buy any edible product with a manufacturing date older than sixty days or thereabouts if there is no expiration date on the label.
2. Pay attention to the way a product is packaged: does it look like professional packaging of food that you find in the grocery store? Packaging is important to maintain integrity of a perishable product like an edible. Check that all packaging and seals are intact.
3. Avoid products with knock-off names of mainstream corporate brands. Not only is this a trademark violation, but the fact that the manufacturer has not taken time to think that through leaves me wondering about what else they haven't thought through. Thankfully, these products are less common in dispensaries than they once were, but they are still around.

4. Be mindful of the way a dispensary stores and displays their edible products. Are they all in a pile, or neatly arranged on clean shelves, or kept in refrigerators for freshness? A sloppy display of edibles is not a good sign that the dispensary practices care and cleanliness with these products.

Herbal Apothecary Products

Tincture: When phytocannabinoids are extracted from cannabis plant material with alcohol, this is called a *tincture*. A tincture is a versatile way to use phytocannabinoids by the dropperful. These products are sometimes made to serve the acidic, raw version of a phytocannabinoid, like CBDA or THCA. Occasionally, these extracts are blended with extracts of other herbs such as turmeric or chamomile to build the desired entourage in order to influence the effect of the final product. They can be taken directly on the tongue or put into a hot beverage. Tinctures may result in a 11 Hydroxy THC experience in your body when they are taken orally.

Tea and tisane: Tea and herbal beverage products are becoming more popular than ever because of their versatility in the way that they can be blended with a variety of herbs to support the entourage effect of the cannabis infusion. Check labels for ingredients and phytocannabinoid content. You may need to portion this product in order to serve yourself a dose that is appropriate for a beginner. These products may result in a 11 Hydroxy THC experience in your body.

Drops / pills / capsules: This product category is one of convenience typically for medical cannabis patients. The product is intended to be used orally and will result in the conversion to 11 Hydroxy THC experience in your body if the product contains delta-9 THC. These products may be blended with other herbs for entourage support. Read the labels to understand the exact dose of phytocannabinoids you will be taking per pill or capsule.

Herbal blends: This product category covers almost everything else apothecary-related: herbal infused oils, sprays, multi-herb and cannabis blends, etc. Each product should be labeled with the phytocannabinoid information so that you can calculate your doses. Depending on the kind of product this is, it may or may not result in a 11 Hydroxy THC experience if it contains THC. Sprays, for example, may not because they are intended to absorb through the mucosal membranes in your mouth and not to be swallowed.

Suppository and intimate products: This is an interesting class of products that always seem to raise eyebrows. Medical cannabis patients are often the consumers of these products, as they provide particular relief for certain symptoms that can't be addressed by other products. They are also enjoyed as a leisure product. I'm not convinced these are a great product for a beginner—certainly not for a first-time cannabis experience. But, if you find that you like other types of apothecary products, you may want to try these, especially if you are a medical cannabis card holder seeking very specific kinds of symptom relief. Read these labels carefully. Sometimes the phytocannabinoid content can be very high for a single serving. Check manufacturing dates, and don't purchase these products if they are more than ninety days old or if the product has a broken seal. Pay close attention to the manner that the dispensary stores and displays this product to ensure its integrity.

Tips for Evaluating Herbal Apothecary Products

1. Make sure that you understand all the ingredients blended into these products. Many of these products sold in dispensaries are blended with other herbs, so it is important to understand what you are purchasing and why.
2. Because some of these products can result in a 11 Hydroxy THC experience, it's very important to calculate dosages carefully based on the amounts stated on the label.
3. Check labeling for manufacturing date and phytocannabinoid content. Because these products often have very specialized formulation, I would not purchase products with manufacturing dates older than three months.

Spa and Topical Products

These products will always be my first choice for a beginner or anyone who is unsure about the kind of cannabis experience they would like to have. I think these products are also great for beginners who are anxious and traumatized by cannabis prohibition propaganda like many in the older generations have been. Most of these products will not result in a psychoactive experience. That's not a guarantee, but in most cases, commercial dispensary spa and topical products do not have enough THC or penetration enhancement to cause any euphoric effect.

Bath bombs and salts: These tend to be a little pricey at dispensaries for what you actually get. Nevertheless, they are a popular product, especially for women. But anyone can enjoy the soothing relief of a hot cannabis-infused bath experience. I don't recommend products in this category that do not disclose ingredients on the labels. By law in most areas, they must disclose phytocannabinoid content and testing, but they do not always have to disclose all of the ingredients.

Lotions / creams / massage oils: Many times, lotions and massage oils will be the best products in this product category that you will find in the dispensary. These products may or may not be high in THC content, but even the products formulated to be high in THC will not cause psychoactive effects. These products are great for sore muscles and workout-related aches and pains.

Salves / balms: Dispensaries will carry various salve formulations, some more well thought out in terms of formulation than others. They can be heavy and greasy depending on how they are formulated. For example, salves formulated with mostly coconut oil (a poor formulation, in my opinion) will tend to be greasier, while formulations with high-oleic-acid oils and MCT oils will be light and absorb quickly. One product in this category that I really like are cannabis-infused lip balms, and I recommend these products for beginners who are already fans of regular lip balm!

Liniment and rubs: These are great products for fast relief. Because they are typically formulated with alcohol, they absorb quickly and provide instant relief. They may have other ingredients, like camphor, which build upon the entourage of the cannabis infusion. They can be dispensed as a roll-on or pump for better dosing options.

Skincare products: There are quite a few strictly skincare brands using phytocannabinoids in their formulations and sold only at dispensaries. So, what is the difference between these and the CBD skin care products sold in retail stores? Retail store products are usually

CBD-isolate products, and they are always made from hemp that is less than 0.30 percent THC hemp by weight. Dispensary skincare products do not have to meet this standard and may contain more THC. Also, dispensary skin care products may be formulated with whole cannabis infusions of novel phytocannabinoids like CBC.

Transdermal patches: There is some debate about how many of these you have to use at once if you want to experience euphoric effects. I've heard reports about these products that vary a lot. They can be expensive products, and they are supposed to deliver phytocannabinoids directly into the bloodstream. I've also had mixed results the times I have tried these products. Since I make all my own spa and topical products, and I have only two recipes that have reliably produced any psychoactivity, these patches have left me wanting more when I have used them. I think, for a beginner, they may be a good product to try—but be aware of the cost in terms of the effects they produce.

Tips for Evaluating Spa and Topical Products

1. Labeling is the first aspect you should evaluate when browsing these products in a dispensary. Quality products will be forthcoming on their labels regarding **all ingredients** contained in the product. This is very important if you have had allergies or sensitivities to any hygiene, topical, or spa product in the past. It is my personal viewpoint that companies who do not disclose ingredients are not operating with the high ethical standards I demand for my topical and spa products.

2. Look for products that are similar to mainstream products you've previously used in terms of supporting ingredients and type of formulation. Always do a small patch test on your arm of any dispensary spa or topical product to ensure you do not have any reaction before applying it over larger parts of your body. Some dispensaries have sample bottles of lotion on the counter that customers can try. Take advantage of this if it is available so you can try the product before you buy it. Dispensaries do not allow customers to return products in most instances.

3. Check labels for manufacturing dates, and don't buy a spa or topical product with a manufacturing date that is more than six months or thereabouts. Sometimes, when

---

dispensary ownership and staff do not understand how to sell topical and spa products to customers, these products will remain on the shelves for months or even a year in that dispensary. And this brings us to the other leg of this issue: When topical and spa products move quickly off the shelf at a dispensary, you can be assured that the dispensary knows how to sell the products to customers, how to store and handle the products appropriately, and that the customer base purchasing these products from that dispensary have had, and continue to have, a good experience with the topical and spa products sold at that dispensary.

4. Sometimes topical and spa products are an afterthought in dispensaries. What do I mean by this? Sometimes dispensary owners and staff don't know very much about this product category and will give the wrong information about using these products and inappropriately store the inventory of these products. It's okay if a dispensary only carries a couple of lotions or only one massage oil. What matters is how these products are being stored and handled in the store. Are all seals intact on the product you are purchasing, or are dispensary staff opening bottles for customers to test or smell that are also for sale to customers? This is more common than you might think. We actually have a long way to go to educate many dispensary owners and staff about topical and spa products. This is not surprising since topicals and spa were unheard of in relation to cannabis over the past ninety years of prohibition.

5. If you are purchasing a topical for the first time, purchase the smallest size they have for sale so you can try it and see how it works for you. Even if a dispensary provides samples from a sample jar or bottle at the counter, it's not like you can put that on your knees or hip joints and really give it a test drive. Buy the smallest size, and if you like it and it works for you, you can always go back for a larger size.

How to Read Product Labels and Check Dates for Freshness

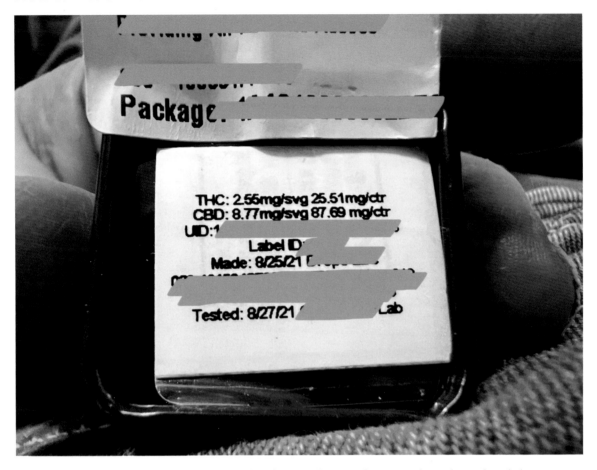

This is an actual product label from a legal cannabis product purchased at a legal dispensary. This label is used to track the product and verify its authenticity and legality. Labels in your legal location will have a similar look. Let's explore and understand each of the elements of this label moving top to bottom:

- the name of the cannabis company who manufactured the product
- lines of product identification numbers for regulation compliance
- phytocannabinoid amounts per serving and per package. This is denoted as svg (serving) and ctr (container)
- more lines of identification numbers for the product
- date of manufacture

- more regulatory numbers related to product, and testing
- full name and address of the manufacturer
- date of testing and the name of the testing lab

Other information, such as product ingredients, is typically found on a second label on the package. Labels can contain very tiny print, so if you have trouble reading product labels, bring a reading or magnification glass with you to use while shopping.

Make a List of Preliminary Product Selections and Budget

Don't worry about memorizing all of these product offerings that you may find at the dispensary! Read through them and make a note about which ones interest you the most. Trying some of the manufactured products is a good first step for beginners to sample a few things and see what they like. Buying raw-flower products will be for those who vaporize, smoke, or want to make their own recipes at home.

Prices vary a lot from location to location. On subsequent visits to the dispensary, you will likely have a budget in mind for each trip. Keep a logbook of the items you want to try, items you've tried, and prices to determine what will fit into your budget. Keep note of when the dispensary offers senior day, veterans' day, or day of the week specials on the product categories you use and enjoy the most. Find out if your favorite dispensary offers a points club for discounts or free items when you spend a certain amount.

Let's Go Guide for Your First Visit

Before going to the dispensary, make sure you have all of the things you'll need to have a satisfying shopping experience. My suggested list of things to prepare in advance are:

1. State or locale-issued ID and, if necessary, your medical cannabis card or medical cannabis recommendation from your doctor and any additional paperwork a dispensary might need to allow you to shop there. All dispensaries have a website that will advise you on what to bring to your visit.
2. Hand sanitizer, mask, and a small package of tissue.

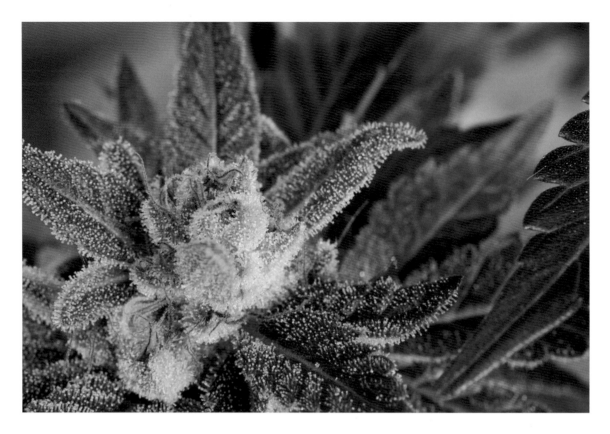

3. Magnifying glass for reading product labels and a jeweler's loupe if you will be purchasing raw cannabis products like flowers. Some of the better dispensaries have nice magnifying apparatuses installed for customers to use but not all do.

4. Cash. Because of conflicts with federal law, it's difficult for dispensaries to offer all banking services to consumers as of the writing of this book. Most dispensaries will want to be paid in cash. Some dispensaries do have ATM machines on-site where you can obtain cash for your visit, but these often have fees to make withdrawals.

5. If you have children or extraordinarily nosy animals in the home, it is suggested that you bring a locking satchel or case that you can put all of your purchases in before leaving the dispensary.

Staff Attitudes and Conduct

As a customer in a dispensary, don't be shy about asking a lot of questions—especially as a first-time customer.

Good service is when the person fulfilling your order is able to clearly understand your needs and recommend the appropriate products. Some dispensary staff are really good at their job, and some are not. It's just like any other service, in fact! If you aren't pleased with how your visit is going, you are under no obligation to make a pity purchase. You can say, "Thank you, I'll be back," or some other variation on this if you would like to explore a different dispensary to compare levels of service and product offerings.

Why the Quality of Information and Guidance at Dispensaries Is All Over the Map

There's really no regulation as to the quality of information you will receive when shopping at a dispensary. Some dispensary owners and staff are adept and are also continually learning and refining their knowledge, and some are stuck in their ways. This isn't so dissimilar to a local health food store. This can be confusing for a beginner, because one staff member will give you some information that is contradicted by another staff member at another dispensary.

When it comes to being a cannabis consumer, medical or leisure, it's up to you to study the information you need to know before your visit. Research information with supporting evidence. Let the person behind the counter do what they do best: serve and explain the products.

Evaluating Sanitary Practices

Look for the signs that a dispensary cares about your health and safety: clean floors, fixtures and counters, staff with clean hands and preferably filling your order using disposable gloves, hand sanitizer for customer use, mask-wearing where required. Are the products fresh and the manufacturing dates within a reasonable window? Cannabis dispensaries will smell like cannabis, but any disagreeable smells like sewage or musty odors should not be present inside.

Home Delivery Services

Many locales where cannabis has legal status for medical or leisure use also have home delivery services. If you would prefer to use these out of a desire for discretion, research these on Google for other customer reviews and for links to websites with menus available for home shopping. I have previously used services like this, and most of the time, the experience was very good. These services are also cash-based and may need to see specific identification or paperwork before they can serve you. Tipping is suggested if the service you are using allows tipping. I have found, in my home delivery experiences, that it will almost always be the same person who delivers an order to my home if I am ordering at the same time every time I order. This will vary, of course, but getting to know your delivery person is a good idea because they will be able to fill you in on everything that is offered, occasionally bring free samples (if this is allowed under state or local law), and alert you about specials and discounts.

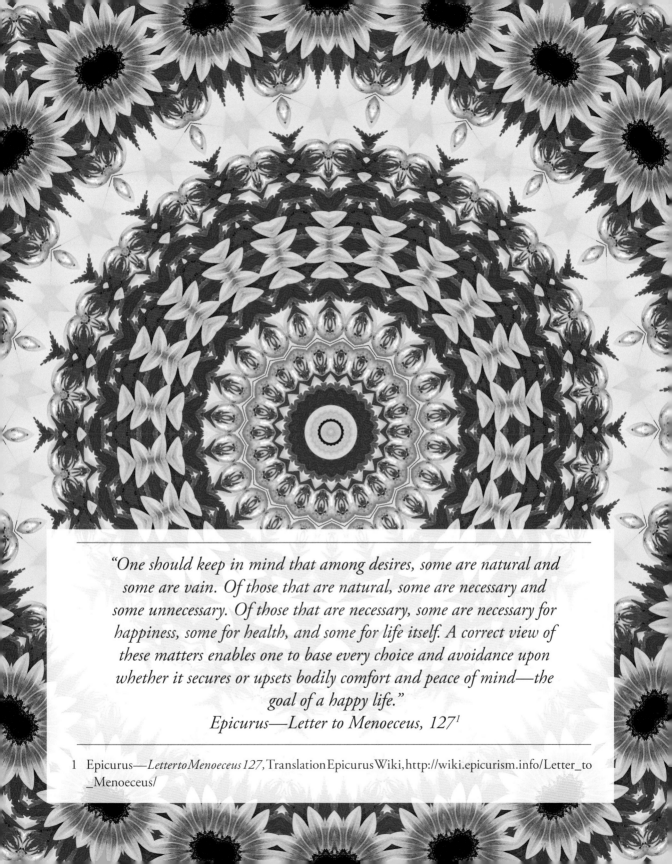

"One should keep in mind that among desires, some are natural and some are vain. Of those that are natural, some are necessary and some unnecessary. Of those that are necessary, some are necessary for happiness, some for health, and some for life itself. A correct view of these matters enables one to base every choice and avoidance upon whether it secures or upsets bodily comfort and peace of mind—the goal of a happy life."

Epicurus—Letter to Menoeceus, 127[1]

1   Epicurus—*Letter to Menoeceus 127*, Translation Epicurus Wiki, http://wiki.epicurism.info/Letter_to _Menoeceus/

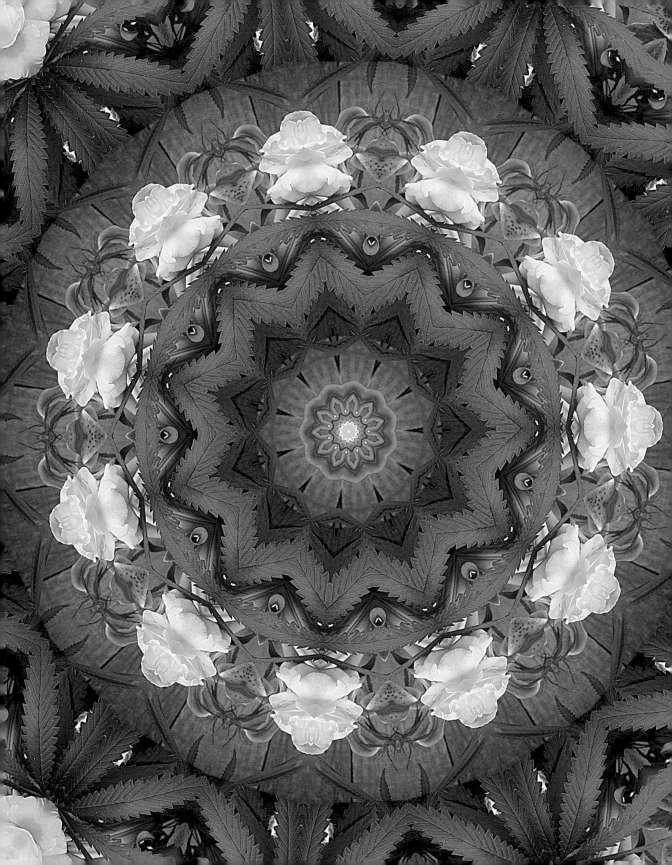

CHAPTER FIVE

LOTIONS AND POTIONS AND SPA TIME: EASY (MOSTLY) TEMPERATE RECIPES FOR YOUR FIRST TIME

As the author who wrote the first modern text to be published about cannabis topicals and spa (The Cannabis Spa at Home, 2015), cannabis spa preparations are my most highly recommended products for a cannabis greenhorn to try for their very first experience with this plant. While many of these products can be a bit pricey and lacking in cannabinoid richness in many of the commercial markets, fortunately, making cannabis topicals and spa preparations at home is one of the simplest, budget-friendly, and foolproof ways to work with cannabis flowers and resins.

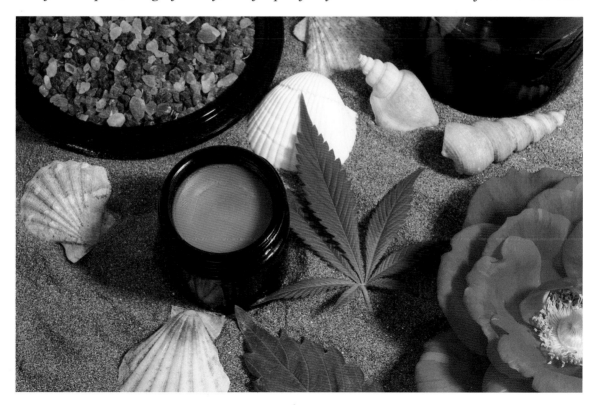

Cannabis Topicals and Spa Basics

In the first chapter of this book, we have touched on the topic of cannabis as a topical and transdermal herbal preparation throughout history. I like to call these "cannabis spa," as that is their most important application in the modern world. In this chapter, you will learn various methods for making cannabis spa preparations at home with a few ingredients, some of which you probably already have in your kitchen cabinet.

Many people find these cannabis spa preparations such as salves, lotions, roll-ons, and baths to be effective for pain and symptom relief without any psychoactive or intoxicating experiences. Indeed, cannabis spa can utilize the power of very high doses of THC in a formulation without the "high" that would normally accompany such doses. Cannabis spa formulation can also utilize many of the other cannabinoids, CBD being the most popular. Many people find that a combination of cannabinoids in a cannabis spa preparation will give them the most satisfying experience. Your individual experience will vary in this regard.

Before you embark upon making these recipes, I suggest you obtain a variety of raw cannabis materials, including flowers that are rich in THC, CBD, and if possible, CBG. THC and CBD will be the most common raw material that you encounter and will be sufficient to get started. As you work through the recipes, try making small batches with each kind of flower and a blend of all the flowers to develop formulations that are right for you.

There are three ways that a cannabis spa formulation can work for you: As a strictly topical formulation (one that is specifically for the skin, like skin healing salves or moisturizers), as a transdermal (one that is formulated with ingredients that facilitate penetration through the skin for applications such as a balm for joint pain or a rub for muscle pain), and as a formula with mucous membrane activity (one that comes into contact with mucous membranes such as a bath preparation or intimate lotion).

For the home spa crafter, but also for professional crafters, it is relevant to note that in clinical research of transdermal drug delivery, olive oil and its compound, oleic acid, is remarkable for the purposes of delivering drugs through the skin for applications such as joint or muscle pain.[1]

---

1 Viljoen, Joe, Amé Cowley, Jan Preeze, Minja Gerber, and Jeanetta Du Plessis. "Penetration enhancing effects of selected natural oils utilized in topical dosage forms." *Drug Development and Industrial Pharmacy.* 2015. 41.2045–2054. 10.3109/03639045.2015.1047847. https://www.researchgate.net/publication/277522269 _Penetration_enhancing_effects_of_selected_natural_oils_utilized_in_topical_dosage_forms

Newer studies in transdermal cannabinoid delivery also note the efficacy of oleic acid and ethanol in this application.[2]

The ingredients we will use as herbal craftspeople to facilitate the work of cannabinoids in a spa formulation will be simple to obtain and easy to work with. We can't duplicate lab results, but we can employ many of the same ingredients that have already been studied to create spa formulations that will be effective for our purposes.

Cannabis Topicals and Spa Myth Busting

Have you heard that cannabinoid-infused topical/transdermal preparations won't get you high and won't cause you to have a positive drug test? **In my opinion, this has been such**

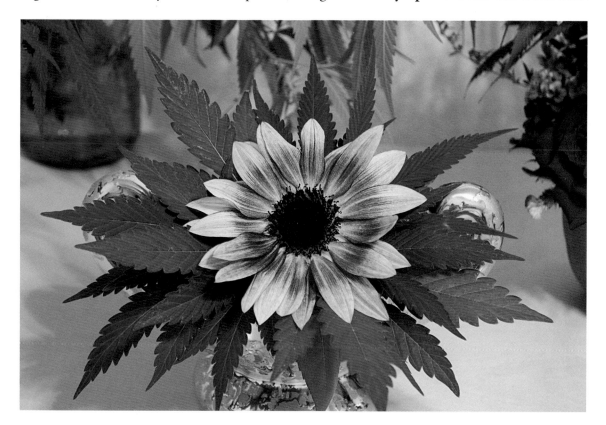

2   Akeemat O. Tijani, Divya Thakur, Dhruv Mishra, Dorcas Frempong, Umeh I. Chukwunyere, Ashana Puri, "Delivering therapeutic cannabinoids via skin: Current state and future perspectives." *Journal of Controlled Release.* 2021. 334. 427–451, ISSN 0168-3659, https://doi.org/10.1016/j.jconrel.2021.05.005 . https://www.sciencedirect.com/science/article/pii/S0168365921002194

an enduring myth because it's actually true in many instances. But . . . it's not always true, and this is why I encourage caution with cannabis spa because it is possible to experience psychoactivity, and you most certainly would not want to use cannabinoid-rich preparations if you have to pass a drug test. Even if what you apply to your skin does not enter your bloodstream, think about all the times we touch mucous membranes like our mouths unconsciously throughout the day. Mucosal absorption of cannabinoids will return a positive drug test, and so will anything that passes through your skin via transdermal absorption—something that's useful if you are using a topical preparation for joint or muscle pain management, but not so useful if you have to take a drug test.

Unless you are using flowers or other raw materials free of THC, you'll always want to apply your topicals and wait at least 2 to 3 hours before doing something like driving or operating dangerous machinery to assess any possible psychoactivity. Many people, including me, prefer spa that is rich in cannabinoids like THC. Many of the topicals that I find most effective for my own needs are very rich in THC. I err on the side of caution with these, and I would encourage you to do the same.

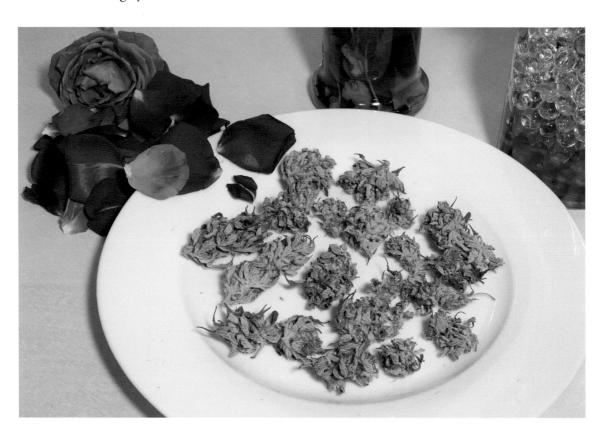

Why Making Is Often Better than Buying

There are quite a few topical and transdermal brands you will encounter in a dispensary. Many of these are good products, and some are not. The real problem with commercial dispensary spa products is the pricing in many cases! You can purchase raw, cured flowers or hashish from the dispensary, and make your own custom topicals and spa for a fraction of the price. And if you grow cannabis at home, you can make topicals and spa for practically free.

Making your own topicals and spa also allows you to experiment with formulation and the construction of an entourage of other herbs or aromatics around the cannabinoids to create what is the most effective for your needs. I can't stress the importance of experimentation enough. I have always written recipes not as a hard rule book on how to make topicals and spa, but to encourage experimentation. And this is the value of crafting custom spa preparations over off-the-shelf purchases at dispensaries: you are in control of every ingredient and can create cannabinoid doses that work best for you.

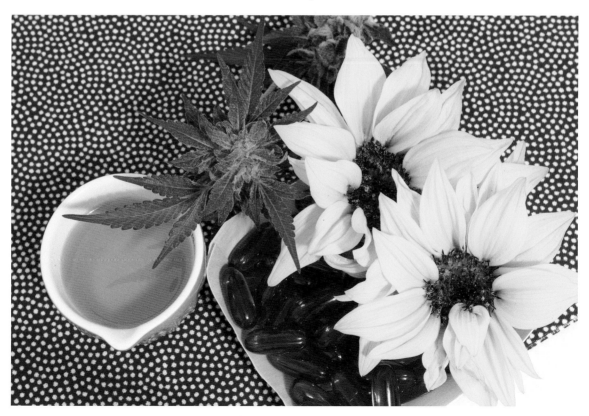

A Beginner's Supply Checklist for Making Salves, Lotions, Baths, and Rubs

Depending on what kinds of cannabis spa products you would like to make, the basic ingredients you keep on hand may be different from this list. This list covers the basic recipes found in this chapter. All of these ingredients are versatile, and I encourage you to experiment with them to make your own custom formulations.

- Aloe vera plant, at least 1 large (live) one (Do not substitute bottled juice. Fresh aloe is necessary for achieving emulsification in some cannabis spa recipes.)
- Beeswax or a vegan alternative like candelilla wax or bayberry myrtle wax
- Camellia tea seed oil (The oil from the seed of camellia; this ingredient can be ordered online if you cannot find it locally.)
- Coarse sea salt
- Cocoa butter
- High-quality olive oil
- Liquid sunflower seed lecithin (Capsules are fine, they can be opened and added to recipes.)
- Soapberries (*Sapindus mukurossi,* these can be ordered online if not available locally.)

Crafting Topicals and Spa with the Entourage Effect

In the first recipe on page 118, you will learn that you can add basic kitchen spices and herbs to the salve recipe to create a warming effect, fragrance, and boost the effects of the cannabinoids. This is the basic principle of an entourage. By using aromatic plants and some other herbs, you can build an entourage around the cannabinoids in a recipe. Many people find that this enhances the cannabis spa experience.

Some ingredient ideas for building entourage:

Basil flowers	Cinnamon bark
Citrus peels	Mint leaf
Frankincense resin	Myrrh resin
Foraged pine or conifer resins	Peppercorns, white or black
Lavender spikes	

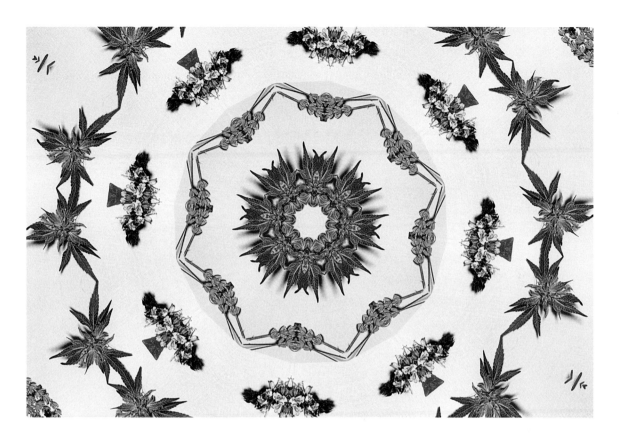

Whole aromatics are preferred when making cannabis spa formulations to create a lighter and fresh fragrance and take advantage of all that a whole herb has to offer. Essential oils may also be used in judicious amounts, but these will only contain terpenes and nothing else from the aromatic plant. The purpose of entourage is not to overpower the fragrance of the cannabis, but rather to complement it so that the final result smells more like a garden and not a perfume factory covering the odor of cannabis.

RECIPES

One-Ingredient Topical Salve

In my first book, *The Cannabis Spa at Home,* I pioneered a method of making a hard cannabis salve with one ingredient: olive oil. In order for this method to work, you need to use very high-quality olive oil: a virgin first cold press olive oil. Sometimes cheap olive oils have been adulterated with other cheaper oils—avoid cheap, generic, or big box brands and look for an olive oil with a

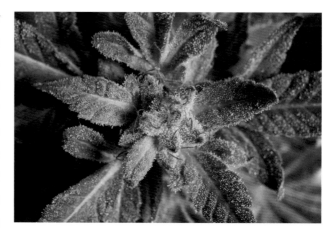

single origin. I prefer California olive oils, and these are pretty easy to find anywhere in the United States.

This salve absorbs quickly and is extremely versatile because it can be used as a base for many other preparations. You can add other warming or soothing herbs or spices from your kitchen cabinet into the recipe if you would like to do that. Try one or more of these: ginger, black pepper, cayenne, cloves, cinnamon, thyme.

This salve is processed in the freezer and stored in the freezer or refrigerator, which will not only keep it at a soothing, cool temperature when it is applied, but it will also remain in a solid state for ease of use.

Makes 1 small batch

Instructions:

Ingredients:

1 cup (240 ml) pure olive oil

3–8 grams cannabis flower of your choice (THC, CBD, CBG or any combination of flowers)

1–3 teaspoons (3–12 grams) of the kitchen spice or herb of your choice*

1. In a double boiler, add all the cannabis and the optional spices to the oil in the top pan and cover. Add water to the bottom pan and process on a medium-low simmer covered on the stove for 90 minutes. Do not let the pan with the water boil to dryness. Add more water as necessary to complete the process. Alternatively, you may want to try a long process in a slow cooker. Add all the

ingredients to the ceramic bowl and cover. Process on low overnight 12 to 18 hours.

2. After processing, allow the oil to cool to room temperature for easy handling.

3. Filter the herbal mixture from the oil using 2 layers of cheesecloth. Squeeze as much of the oil out of the herbs as you can.

4. Pour the oil into the final salve container you would like to use. Your container should be clean and sanitized.

5. Place the salve container with the oil in the freezer. This will completely harden in about 60 to 90 minutes. Once it is completely hardened, you can use the salve.

6. Store the salve in the freezer or refrigerator and use as needed. Use within 2 months for best results.

---

* Some great ideas for this are warming spices like cinnamon, pepper, clove, and ginger, but you can use any kitchen herb or spice that you prefer.

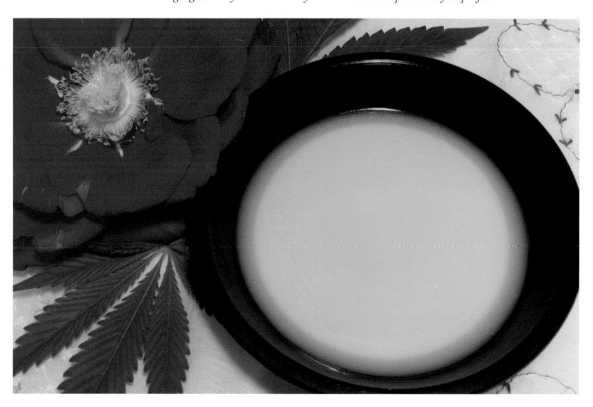

Easy Resinous Cannabis Roll-Ons

This recipe is a great example of why you may want to use whole aromatic herbs instead of essential oils in your spa recipes. This recipe uses whole frankincense resin. The whole resin of frankincense contains boswellic acid, which is not in the essential oil of frankincense. The boswellic acid molecule is too large to pass through the distillation process used to make essential oils along with many of the other compounds in the raw frankincense resin. Boswellic acid is essential to obtain benefits from frankincense, because it is boswellic acid that has been identified in research as the compound responsible for the anti-inflammatory effects of frankincense.[3]

This roll on can be used for muscle pain, shoulder pain, or back and joint pain. It also makes a soothing roll-on for irritated or dry skin.

Makes several bottles of roll-ons, depending on chosen size

Instructions:

1. In a double boiler, add the oil, cannabis flowers, frankincense, and sunflower lecithin to the top pan and cover. Add water to the bottom pan and process on a medium-low simmer covered on the stove for 60 minutes, stirring frequently. Do not let the pan with the water boil to dryness. Add more water as necessary to complete the process.

2. After the mixture is finished processing, you may notice that there is frankincense resin remaining undissolved. This is normal; this is the water-soluble compound from the resin. It will not dissolve in the oil and will be discarded.

Ingredients:
- 1 cup (240 ml) olive oil or camellia tea seed oil
- 3–8 grams of cannabis flower of your choice (THC, CBD, CBG or any combination of flowers)
- 20 grams frankincense resin
- 1 teaspoon (5 ml) liquid sunflower lecithin

---

3 Farah Iram, Shah Alam Khan, and Asif Husain, "Phytochemistry and potential therapeutic actions of boswellic acids: A mini-review," *Asian Pacific Journal of Tropical Biomedicine*, vol. 7, no. 6, 2017, 513–523, ISSN 2221-1691, https://doi.org/10.1016/j.apjtb.2017.05.001. https://www.sciencedirect.com/science/article/pii/S2221169117304914

3. As soon as the mixture cools enough to safely handle, filter the herbal mixture from the oil using two layers of cheesecloth. Squeeze as much of the oil out of the herbs as you can.

4. Stir the oil and then fill the clean, sanitized roller ball bottles, and affix the roller tops and lids. Amber or Miron glass roller bottles are suggested to maintain freshness.

5. Store unopened and unused bottles in a cool, dark area until you are ready to use them. Use these bottles within 3 months.

Oranges and Spice Cannabis Lip Balm

Lip balm is a big favorite of many of the readers of my other recipe books, so including a really yummy one here that's also easy to make is a no-brainer! This lip balm recipe has orange and spice flavors that everyone loves, and also has a bit of chocolate flavor from the cocoa butter that just goes so well with the orange and spice.

Makes several lip balms, depending on size of containers chosen

Instructions:

1. In a small pan on the stove, or in the microwave, gently melt together the cacao butter, olive oil, beeswax, liquid sunflower lecithin, and the full-extract cannabis oil.

2. After melting and combining, add the essential oils and stir. Pour the lip balm into clean, sanitized balm containers.

3. Process in the freezer until hard. The lip balm will soften a little after being removed from the freezer. Don't skip this step, because the freezing process will ensure a smooth lip balm free of all graininess.

4. Store unused lip balm in a cool, dark cabinet. Use all the lip balm within 3 months.

Ingredients:
¼ cup (60 ml) cacao butter
2 tablespoons (30 ml) olive oil
1 tablespoon (15 ml) beeswax
1 teaspoon (5 ml) liquid sunflower lecithin
1 teaspoon (5 ml) full-extract cannabis oil (RSO is another name for this oil)
10 drops sweet orange essential oil
2 drops cinnamon essential oil
1 drop clove essential oil

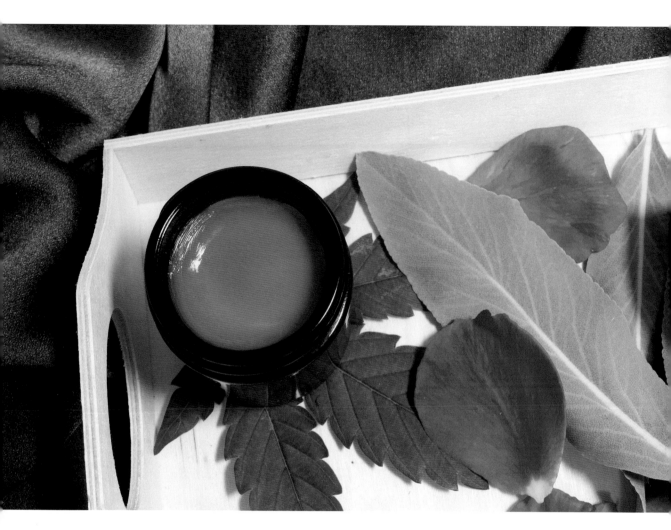

White Sage and Roses Cannabis Salve

This year, I grew white sage in my garden for the first time. I've also got eleven rose bushes in my garden. These two plants really complemented each other; I loved the floral richness of the roses and the camphor fragrance of the sage when I decided to bring them together in a cannabis salve. This is another one of those warming salves, so I think you are really going to enjoy using this for sore muscles and backs.

Makes 1 salve

Instructions:

1. Fill a canning jar with the part measures of all the herbs. You may fill it with as much or as little as you desire, but don't fill it with herbs all the way—leave sufficient room for the oil.

2. Once the jar is full, gently push the herbs down to the bottom. Fill with olive oil just until the herbs are completely covered.

3. Affix the lid and put it in a pan of water with a platform at the bottom of the pan to ensure the jar does not touch the bottom during the heat process, such as a canning boiler.

4. Process on a simmer (medium-low heat) for 90 minutes. Remove from the stove and allow the jar to cool completely inside the pan of water.

5. Remove the jar from the pan and shake. Decant the oil and strain through at least two layers of cheesecloth.

6. Measure the final amount of oil that you have. Add the wax to measure approximately ¾ the amount of the oil, and add 1 teaspoon (5 ml) of liquid sunflower lecithin for each ½ cup (120 ml) of oil and wax combined. Add all of this to a double boiler and process on medium low, stirring frequently until everything melts and is thoroughly combined.

7. Remove from the stove and pour into a clean, sanitized salve jar. Process in the freezer until solid to make a smooth salve free of graininess. Store at room temperature and use within 3 months for best results.

Ingredients:
By weight:
1 part dried white sage
1 part cannabis flowers
2 parts rosebuds and petals

olive oil *(see instructions)*
liquid sunflower lecithin *(see instructions)*
Bayberry wax (or beeswax or candelilla wax) *(see instructions)*

I Got High on Cannabis Topical: A True Story and the Recipe for the Adventurous!

This recipe comes with my biggest caveat: It's for the purposes of obtaining euphoric effects that, quite frankly, can be very helpful for pain relief, in my experience. I can't guarantee you will have the same experience I had with this massage oil, but I can give you the recipe I used and you can decide what you think! This is a recipe you will want to try only on the days you don't need to drive.

My other caveat for this recipe is that you try a small patch test to ensure that you aren't going to be sensitive to Olbas Oil, which is one of the ingredients in this recipe.

I originally made this concentrated oil a couple of years ago to use as single drops in a cup of tea (minus the Olbas Oil). One morning, I woke up with especially excruciating hip pain and happened to have the oil in my room, and because I had no other topicals on hand, I decided to use this oil that I had originally prepared for use in hot beverages. I added some drops of Olbas Oil, just to create a warming sensation, and applied 1 teaspoon or so (5 to 8 ml), allowed it to absorb, and then turned over and applied to the other hip. I closed my eyes and dozed for a bit before waking to a familiar, funny feeling. I was definitely high. I've also been able to duplicate my experience several times using this same oil. It was very effective for the hip pain, too. I don't hesitate to use it if I need to. I can't explain why this recipe affects me this way. Perhaps the location of my hips is more apt to absorb the oil, the high oleic acid content of the camellia seed oil combined with the camphorous essential oil, and the high concentration of THC in the recipe?

This uses camellia tea seed oil, which is a specialty oil that you may not find locally, but a small bottle can be ordered for a reasonable price online. It's essential if you want to try to duplicate my results. The other ingredient is an essential oil blend called Olbas Oil. This is a Swiss essential oil blend product that is available in most natural food stores, or it can be ordered easily online. Olbas oil blends many camphorous aromatics, including wintergreen and peppermint, which makes this a very warming and soothing oil. Don't substitute anything else if you would like to try to duplicate my results. Feel free to double this recipe if you would like to make more to fill a larger bottle suitable for massage oils.

Makes 2 ounces (60 ml)

Instructions:

1. Fill a small canning jar such as a small jam or jelly jar with the oil and hashish.
2. Affix the lid and put it in a pan of water with a platform at the bottom of the pan to ensure the jar does not touch the bottom during the heat process, such as a canning boiler.
3. Process on a simmer (medium-low heat) for 90 minutes. Remove from the stove and allow the jar to cool completely inside the pan of water.
4. Depending on the quality of the hashish you have used, there may be a slight amount of plant material remaining; there is no need to strain this out to use this oil.
5. As soon as the mixture cools enough to safely handle, fill the clean, sanitized bottle that you want to store your massage oil in. Add the Olbas Oil and shake. Affix the lid, store in a cool cabinet, and use it within 3 months.

Ingredients:
¼ cup (60 ml) camellia tea seed oil
4 grams (approximately) of any high-THC concentrate such as live rosin or hashish*
½ teaspoon (2.5 ml) liquid sunflower lecithin
15 drops Olbas Oil essential oil

This recipe was originally developed for hip pain, and that seems to be the best place to apply if you want to try to duplicate my results. But you can also apply it to your knees or other joints if you prefer.

---

* *The total THC in this recipe should be around 1600 to 2000 mg of THC. Dispensary hashish products will have the exact milligrams on the label, which should make this easier!*

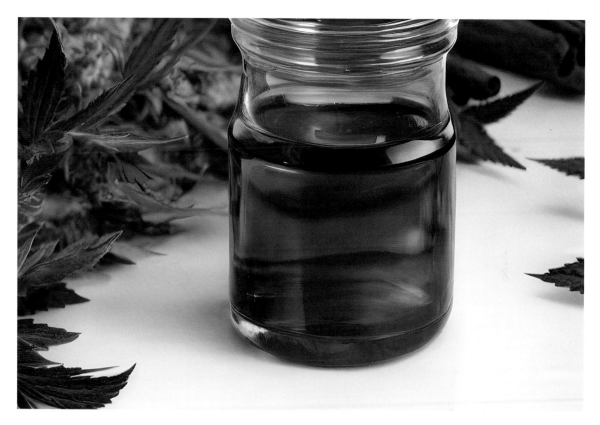

Kaneh Bosem, the Biblical Anointing Oil

It's impossible to know the exact measure of herbs specified in Exodus for the priestly holy anointing oil recipe, but we can make a close approximation that I am sure you will find fragrant and enlightening. We will prepare this recipe according to the instruction found in scripture to prepare it as a compounded perfume of the finest quality, which at that time meant using a gentle heat to blend the oils and resins from all of the whole herbs included in the recipe. Use this oil for your own private spiritual healing practice or as a simple, warming, anti-inflammatory pain relief massage oil.

Makes a varying amount of oil, depending on how much herbal material you use

Instructions:

1. Fill a canning jar with the part measures of all the herbs. You may fill it with as much or as little as you desire, but don't fill it with herbs all the way—leave sufficient room for the oil.

2. Once the jar is full, gently tap it on the counter to settle the herbs. Fill with olive oil just until the herbs are completely covered.

3. Affix the lid, and put it in a pan of water with a platform at the bottom of the pan to ensure the jar does not touch the bottom during the heat process, such as a canning boiler.

4. Process on a simmer (medium-low heat) for 90 minutes. Remove from the stove and allow the jar to cool completely inside the pan of water.

5. Remove the jar from the pan and shake. Decant the oil and strain through at least two layers of cheesecloth.

6. Pour the oil into a clean, sanitized bottle. You may add some whole myrrh resin chunks, a cannabis flower, a cinnamon stick, and some cassia buds to the bottle for aesthetic appeal. Your anointing oil is ready to use. Store at room temperature and use within 3 months for best results.

Ingredients:
By weight
2 parts myrrh resin
2 parts dried cassia flower buds
1 parts cinnamon bark (specifically *Cinnamomum verum* or Ceylon)
1 part cannabis flower
Olive oil *(see instructions)*

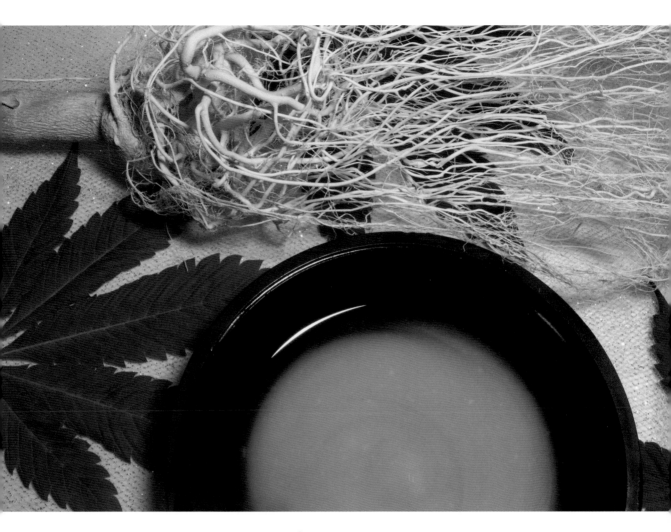

Rootworking Salve

This recipe uses cannabis root—something that you'll definitely have on hand when you grow your first cannabis plant! Don't compost the root; carefully scrub it clean and remove any root hairs that you can't scrub totally clean. Lay it aside in a clean, dry area and allow it to wilt for two days. Chop up the root and allow it to dry out another day. Alternatively, you can use roots that have been dried and chopped for this recipe. I think the fresh root is better, but you can try both dried and fresh together, too!

Cannabis root does not contain cannabinoids. This recipe will give you the opportunity to experience another soothing medicinal property of the cannabis that is totally different from the cannabinoids on the top parts of the plant.

Makes about 7 ounces (225 ml) of salve

Instructions:

Ingredients:
½ cup (120 ml) olive oil
1 whole cannabis root, chopped and dried
⅓ cup + 1 tablespoon (95 ml) beeswax or vegan wax like cadellia or bayberry
2 teaspoons (10 ml) liquid sunflower lecithin
Optional: 1–3 drops rosemary essential oil

1. In a double boiler, add the olive oil and the cannabis root to the top pan and cover. Add water to the bottom pan and process on a medium-low simmer on the stove for 60 minutes, stirring frequently. Do not let the pan with the water boil to dryness. Add more water as necessary to complete the process.

2. After the mixture is finished processing, allow this to cool to room temperature and then strain the cannabis root from the oil.

3. Put the oil back into the double boiler along with the beeswax and sunflower lecithin. Heat on medium-low until everything melts, stirring frequently.

4. Remove from the heat and allow to cool briefly, but don't allow it to harden. Pour into a clean, sanitized jar. Add the essential oil, if desired, and stir.

5. Process in the freezer until hard. It will soften after being removed from the freezer and can then be used immediately. The advantage of processing the salve in the freezer as the last step will ensure that your salve is smooth and free of graininess. Use within 2 months for best results.

The Flying Nun Splash and Healing Rub

This is an advanced recipe only because it uses fresh cannabis flowers. You will need to grow these yourself, or perhaps a friend can gift you some! This recipe takes advantage of cannabis resins in their raw state—so what you will experience are cannabinoids like THCA, CBDA, and CBGA. As long as this is kept away from heat and light in a cool, dark cabinet, it should stay fairly stable for at least three months. Aging isn't a bad thing; it's just going to change the cannabinoids over time as they lose carbon atoms to become THC, CBD, CBG, and CBN. Initially, though, if you use this quickly and take care of its storage needs, you should be able to get the nonpsychoactive benefits of the acidic raw cannabinoids.

This recipe is both topical and edible. It makes a great rub, but it's also a tasty tincture that is great for nonpsychoactive relaxation. I prefer this as a cooling rub for hot flashes and sore muscles.

This recipe is based on a recipe from the Middle Ages known as Carmelite water, originally made by the Carmelite nuns. Carmelite water was used for all kinds of things back then. It's interesting to note that colognes were once used both internally and externally for their health benefits. These old-fashioned colognes smell and taste wonderful, unlike if you tried to drink a bottle of modern cologne. They are essentially aromatized tinctures, and that is what this recipe is: an aromatized tincture.

The primary ingredient of Carmelite water was Melissa, otherwise known as lemon balm. The recipe was and still is a guarded secret, but lemon balm forms the basis of the recipe. In my Flying Nun version of this recipe, lemon balm and cannabis are the foundation of the recipe with the addition of supporting herbs and spices.

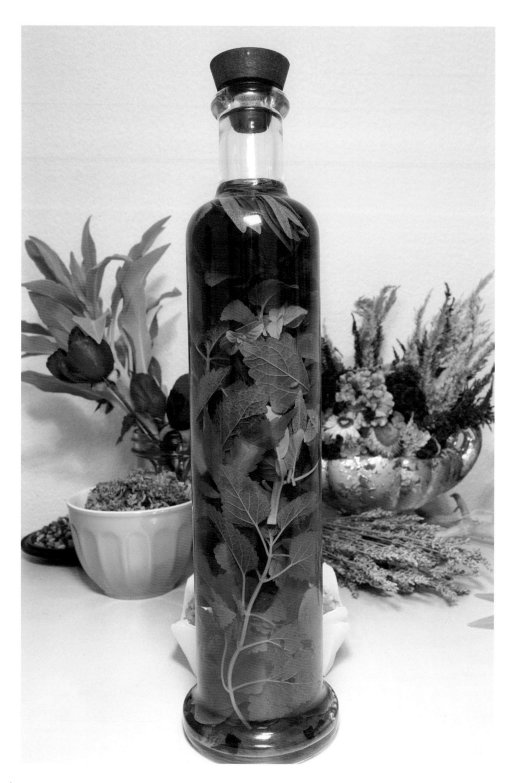

Makes approximately ⅔ of a liter, depending on the amount of herbs used

Ingredients:
1 (750 ml–1 L) glass bottle of 100 to 150 proof vodka*
1 bunch fresh Melissa (lemon balm)
3–5 large, fresh cannabis flowers, or the equivalent in smaller flowers
Peels from 2 large lemons and 1 orange, minus the white pith**
2 sticks cinnamon
½ teaspoon (0.5 g) grated whole nutmeg
1 tablespoon (3 g) whole angelica seeds

Instructions:

1. Pour half of the vodka from the bottle into a measuring cup.
2. Wash the lemon balm and allow it to dry. Add it to the now half-empty bottle of vodka along with the fresh cannabis flowers and all the other ingredients. Use a chopstick or other clean wooden utensil to arrange the herbs in the bottle so that they are as evenly spaced as possible.
3. After you have added all the herbs and arranged them in the bottle, pour the vodka from the measuring cup into the bottle until all of the herbs are completely covered. You will probably have some vodka left over since the herbs will displace the liquid. Store the leftover vodka in a separate bottle, and you can use it later to top up your Flying Nun Splash as you use it.
4. Place the bottle in a cool, dark cabinet and allow it to process for at least 2 weeks. I find that 4 weeks is optimum for this recipe, but it's definitely good after just 2 weeks. Shake the bottle every few days while it's processing.
5. When you are ready to use this, you don't need to decant it, you can use it straight from the bottle! Keep the bottle sealed and in a cool, dark area until you have used the entire mixture. Feel free to top up with more of the leftover vodka as you go, and you can even add more cannabis and lemon balm as needed.
6. Rub on the body, temples, head, and neck. The Flying Nun Splash is great for headaches and stress. If you would like to try some as a tincture, add a dropperful to hot tea or another hot beverage for psychoactive effects or to a cold beverage for non-psychoactive effects.

*The vodka must be 100 proof or greater to sufficiently tincture all of the ingredients.
**Using a potato peeler is the best way to get these peels without including the white pith.

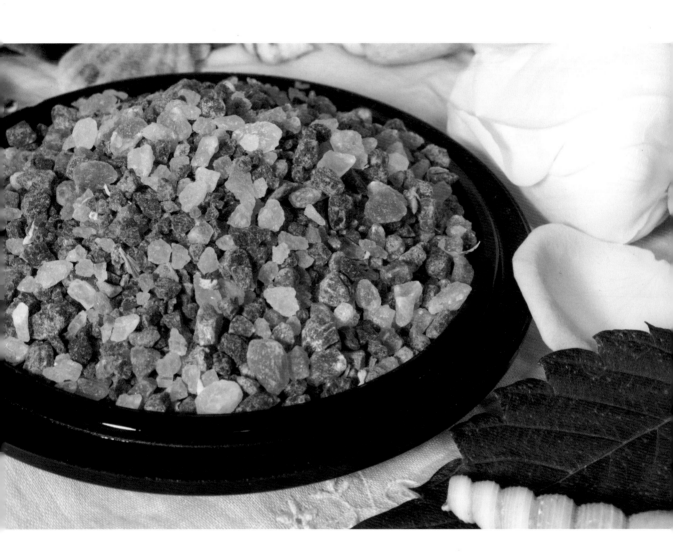

Cannabis-Infused Bath Salts

When I wrote my first cannabis book, *The Cannabis Spa at Home,* I pioneered a method of creating cannabis-infused bath salts using all plant-based ingredients to achieve emulsification of oil in the bath. The results are nothing less than spectacular. This bath is very soft and distributes the oil evenly throughout the water with no ring around the tub.

And, yes, it's possible to experience euphoria from this bath depending on the amount of cannabinoids that are in the water and how long you remain soaking in the bath. **Because this is a bath preparation, cannabinoids will come in contact with mucous membranes and the skin covering most of the body, and this is why it's important to wait at least two hours to ascertain the psychoactivity of the bath before driving.**

You may add less than the amount of the suggested amount of full-extract cannabis oil here if you prefer. This recipe is a variation of the recipe found in my first book, but it is scaled down a bit here to have fewer steps in order to be more beginner friendly.

Makes 2 pounds (1 kg)

Ingredients:

2 cups (480 ml) water
½ cup (120 ml) gel scraped from fresh aloe vera leaves (don't substitute bottled juice or gel)
50 whole soapberries, split and de-seeded (*Sapindus mukorossi* or *Sapindus drummondii*)
2 teaspoons (10 ml) olive oil
1 tablespoon (15 ml) full-extract cannabis oil (also known as RSO)
½ teaspoon (2.5 ml) sunflower lecithin
Assorted essential oils of your preference
2 pounds (1000 g) of large coarse salt crystals (pink or sea salt)

Instructions:

1. In a blender, blend the water and aloe together until smooth, with no chunks remaining. Add this water to a pan on the stove along with the soapberries.

2. Simmer on medium low until the water has thickened and reduced to about ⅔ cup (160 ml) of liquid.

3. While the soapberry mixture is simmering, fully combine the olive oil, full-extract cannabis oil, and the liquid sunflower lecithin in a cup.

4. When the soapberry mixture has reduced to a thickened liquid, remove from the stove and separate the spent berries from the liquid using a strainer.

5. Add the cannabis oil mixture to the warm soapberry mixture and combine thoroughly.

6. Add all the salt to a large bowl and stir in the cannabis-soapberry mixture until it is distributed evenly throughout the salt.

7. Spread the salt on a large baking sheet or on a dehydrator pan lined with parchment paper. Dehydrate the salt mixture in a dehydrator using the heat setting, or in the oven on 200°F (94°C) until the salt absorbs the liquid and is completely dry.

8. Remove from the oven or dehydrator, and spoon the bath salt into a clean, sanitized jar. Add the essential oils of your choice for aromatherapeutic benefits during your bath. Combine thoroughly and store the jar in a cool, dark cabinet. Add a silica moisture absorbing packet if desired. Sometimes a moisture-absorbing pack is helpful for keeping the salt dry if you live in a humid environment.

9. Use ½ cup (225–250 g) to 1 cup (450–500 g) of salt per bath. You can use more or less depending on your preferences or the size of your tub. My suggested amount is sufficient for most soaking tubs. Use the bath salts within 3 months.

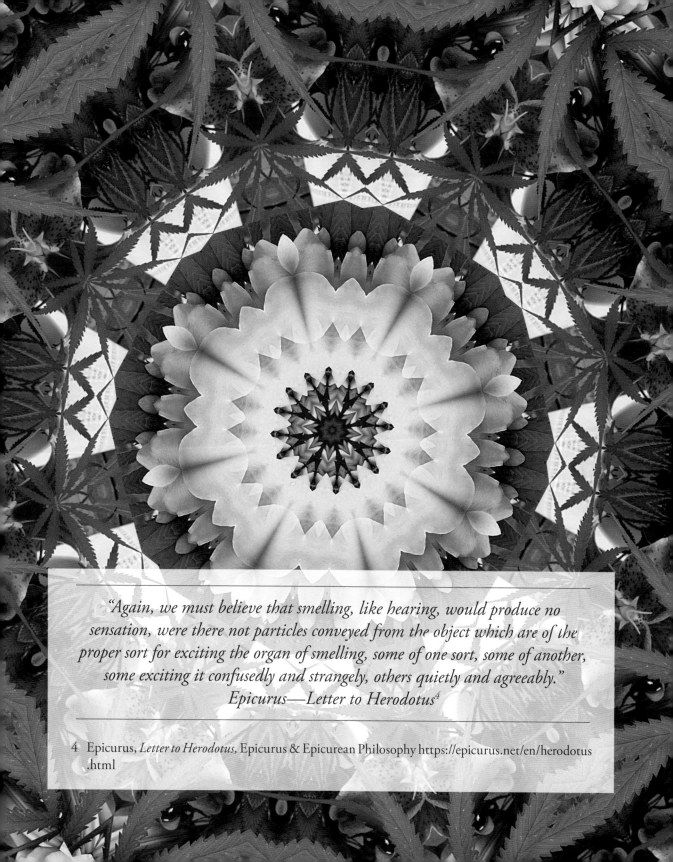

"*Again, we must believe that smelling, like hearing, would produce no sensation, were there not particles conveyed from the object which are of the proper sort for exciting the organ of smelling, some of one sort, some of another, some exciting it confusedly and strangely, others quietly and agreeably.*"
Epicurus—Letter to Herodotus[4]

4   Epicurus, *Letter to Herodotus,* Epicurus & Epicurean Philosophy https://epicurus.net/en/herodotus.html

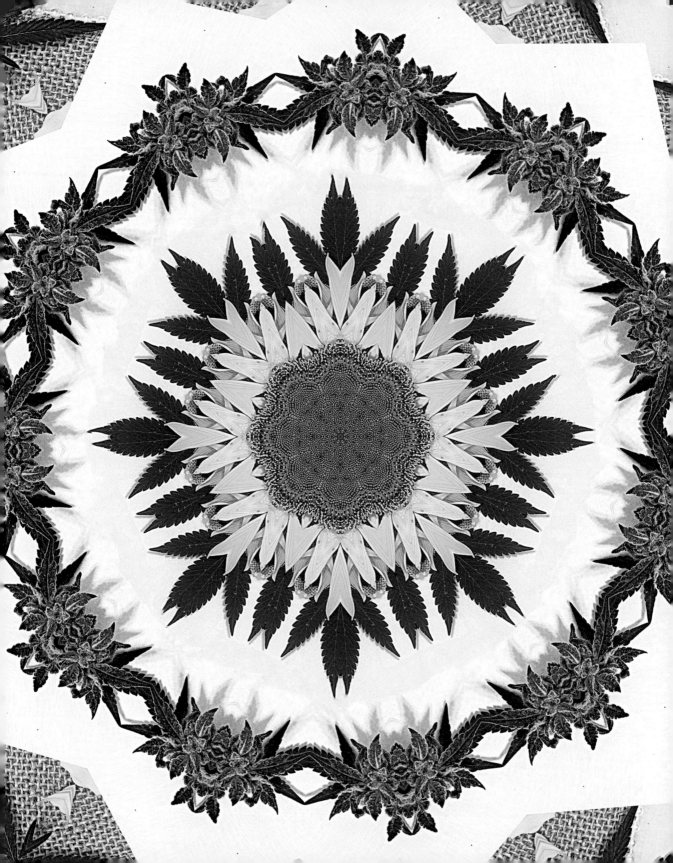

TINCTURES, OILS, MEDICINALS, BEVERAGES, AND EDIBLES: BUILD SIMPLE RECIPES WITH A SOLID FOUNDATION OF BASIC TECHNIQUES

Making organic solvent extracts of cannabis is much easier than it sounds and very budget friendly. Whether you are interested in preparing herbal tinctures, beverages, or medicinals or want to try edibles like cookies, brownies, or gummies, in this chapter, you will learn the basics you need to get started right away making high-quality cannabis extractions.

Cannabinoid Extraction Basics

Cannabinoids are hydrophobic, which means they don't extract into water. They are an oily resin that, at best, will float on top of the water or stick to the sides of a container if mixed with water. In order for cannabinoids to extract, you must use a solvent like alcohol or fat.

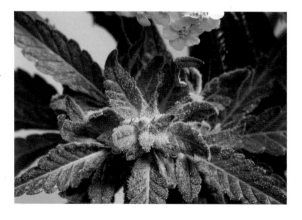

The alcohol concentration has to be strong enough to extract all of the cannabinoids it comes into contact with, and for this reason, I suggest working with only higher proofs of alcohol in order to make cannabis extractions.

When it comes to oils, any oil will do, of course, but according to some research, at least, some oils are a little bit better at performing cannabinoid extraction from raw cannabis material. One such chemistry study that I am fond of sending to the readers of my books who write to me to inquire about what is the "best" oil to use shows evidence for the efficacy of olive oil in extracting cannabinoids.[1]

In personal preparation and in the favorite oil extractions of some of my farmer friends, MCT oil is also a superior oil for cannabinoid extraction, and it lends itself nicely to capturing many of the terpenes, as well. MCT oil is preferred over pure coconut oil, as it has a longer shelf life and has a neutral fragrance.

Solid fats like clarified butter are recommended over plain butter. Plain butter contains some milk protein that can turn rancid. Clarified butter is very shelf-stable and has a long shelf life. Cocoa butter is another favorite of mine as a base for both topicals and edibles. Specialty oils like tea seed and rice bran oil are also good.

Cannabinoid Calculation Basics

Calculation isn't as daunting as it may seem at first, but keep in mind that it is **absolutely critical for decarboxylated edible cannabis recipes** in particular.

You will need an accurate gram scale to work with raw cannabis products in your kitchen.

If you purchase raw cannabis products like flower, trim, or concentrates from a dispensary, calculations for recipes are going to be very easy and will look like this:

1 gram = 1000 mg

1 gram of cannabis flower with 20% THC and 2% CBD
1000 × 20% = 200 mg THC
1000 × 2% = 20 mg CBD

If we use this gram of cannabis flower in these recipes, the calculations are:
1 pan of brownies (12 servings)
200 mg / 12 servings = 16.6 mg THC per serving
20 mg / 12 servings = 1.6 mg CBD per serving

---

1 Romano, L. L., and Arno Hazekamp. "Cannabis oil: Chemical evaluation of an upcoming cannabis-based medicine." *Cannabinoids*. 2013. 1. 1-11 http://www.cannabis-med.org/data/pdf/en_2013_01_1.pdf

*Beginner-sized servings might look like this:

1 pan of brownies (48 bite-sized servings)

200 mg / 48 servings = 4.1 mg THC per serving

20 mg / 48 servings = 0.42 mg CBD per serving

1 mold pan of gummies (30 servings)

200 mg / 30 servings = 6.6 mg THC per gummy

20 mg / 30 servings = 0.6 mg CBD per gummy

Now let's try this with 1 gram of hashish with 45% THC and 15% CBD

$1000 \times 45\% = 450$ mg THC

$1000 \times 15\% = 150$ mg CBD

If we use the entire gram in a recipe the calculations will look like this:

1 sheet of cookies (24 servings)

450 mg / 24 servings = 18.75 mg THC per cookie

150 mg / 24 servings = 6.25 mg CBD per cookie

For the most accurate calculations, always begin with 1 gram, convert to 1000 mg, and multiply by the percentage of cannabinoid in the gram.

For raw cannabis products labeled with the milligrams in each gram instead of the percentage, the calculation is even easier! For 1 gram of product with 170 mg of THC, simply divide into the number of servings (no need to multiply a percentage to get the exact milligrams of each serving):

A pan of 12 brownies using 1 gram of cannabis flower containing 170 mg total THC = 170 / 12 = 14.16 mg THC per brownie

For beginners who are making edibles and other cannabinoid containing recipes, it is always suggested to purchase raw cannabis products from a dispensary that have been tested for the exact amount of cannabinoid in the product to ensure very exact calculations for your edible recipes.

There will be some cannabinoid loss through the decarb process. Professional opinions on this vary. Because cannabis edibles and 11 Hydroxy THC are more intense than the delta-9

THC experience, your calculations will be based on the stated percentage or milligrams on the dispensary product. Remember that if you aren't satisfied, you can always consume more after two hours from your first dose.

If you want to try your hand at growing your own cannabis and using your homegrown cannabis in edible recipes (a bit more advanced, so you are not going to want to do this as the very first edible recipe that you make), you may want to try my personal method for cannabinoid estimation for raw cannabis products that have not been tested for the exact amount of cannabinoids.

This will require some experience with cannabis. As a general rule of thumb, the way this works is that 1 gram of flower is weighed out, and then, based on what my experience is with the smoked or vaporized flower, I will make calculations that look like this:

A small portion of the flower is ground and placed in a glass pipe or a vaporizer. I smoke or vape the portion and see how I feel. If I feel just the right psychoactivity that is comfortable for me, I will weigh the rest of the unused gram and then make a calculation of how many servings are going to be appropriate for me. **Keep in mind that smoking and vaping are mostly delta-9 THC experiences, not the more powerful 11 Hydroxy THC experience of an edible, so calculations of serving sizes need to be predicated on this knowledge.**

Let's assume the following for our gram of homegrown cannabis flower:

After being satisfied with the vape experience with a portion of the 1 gram of flower, the leftover flower from the 1 gram is reweighed and returns a weight of 0.90 gram. So 0.10 gram was the amount I vaped and was satisfied with. Now, for my edible, I will cut this in half to compensate for the more powerful effects of 11 Hydroxy THC, so 0.05 gram will be my benchmark to calculate the number of servings. For the recipe that we intend to use this 1 gram of homegrown cannabis flower for, we will have approximately 20 individual servings. A pan of brownies will need to be sliced into 20 servings.

But what if my homegrown is a "CBD only" plant? Do I need to worry about any psychoactive effects from using these in an edible?

The short answer is YES. Caution rules the day with homegrown "CBD only" plants. Depending on many factors, these plants can, and have, produced THC in percentages that may cause psychoactive effects.

Conducting a test, via vaporizer or by smoking, will help you determine the effects of your cured CBD homegrown. If few or no psychoactive effects are noted, then you may proceed using the same estimation method as you do for THC or THC and CBD combined.

Alcohol Extracts for Tinctures and Beverages

Nonpsychoactive Alcohol Extraction for Tinctures and Beverages

Tinctures are an excellent way to customize cannabinoid content for use straight from the dropper or in a beverage. For those who enjoy the nonpsychoactive, raw acidic cannabinoids THCA and CBDA, tincturing in alcohol is the easiest way to capture and preserve these cannabinoids. To retain them in this state, your cannabis material should be fresh (I suggest homegrown fresh flowers for this).

You will need:
fresh cannabis flowers
canning jars (amber glass is suggested)
120–190 proof culinary grade ethyl alcohol
cheesecloth
glass measuring cup
funnel
amber bottles with droppers for packaging

Instructions:

1. Chop the cannabis flowers and put them in a clean, glass canning jar.
2. Pour alcohol over them, and then push them down a little until the alcohol covers them completely. Use a little more alcohol to accomplish this, if necessary.
3. Affix the lid and put the jar in a cool, dark cabinet for at least 2 weeks. Shake the jar occasionally during that time.
4. Decant the tincture and filter through cheesecloth into a large glass measuring cup. Using a funnel, fill the clean, sanitized dropper bottles and affix the lids. Label each one with the contents.
5. Store in a cool, dark cabinet and **do not expose to light, heat, or air** in order to maintain the integrity of the THCA, CBDA, or other raw acidic cannabinoid. Use these tinctures quickly, within 3 months, for best results.

Many times, when I make these types of tinctures, I will store them in a closed container in the refrigerator.

You may use these tinctures in cold beverages only or take them orally. **Do not use them in hot beverages or on hot food** as it may decarboxylate the cannabinoids. Always shake tinctures before dispensing a serving. Test these by ingesting only a few drops at a time before ingesting a whole dropperful.

Decarbed Psychoactive Alcohol Extraction for Tinctures and Beverages

Making decarboxylated tinctures, such as THC, CBD, or CBG, is similar to making them with oil, and we will use a very similar simple calculation method for both tested raw cannabis dispensary products and homegrown cannabis products that we use for any other recipe.

Instructions:

You will need:
Lab-tested raw cannabis flowers from the dispensary
a small baking dish
120–190 proof culinary grade ethyl alcohol
canning jars (amber glass is suggested)
cheesecloth
glass measuring cup
funnel
amber bottles with droppers for packaging

1. Calculate how many and what size tinctures you would like to make. Weigh the cured cannabis flowers on the gram scale and note the weight. Make a note of either the percentage of cannabinoids in the flowers, or the milligrams of cannabinoids indicated on the label of the product and the total weight of the plant material.

   Before doing anything, make your calculation. Let's look at this example calculation for 3 grams of 20% THC and 5% CBD raw flower:

   3 grams = 3000 milligrams total weight
   + 4 ounces (120 ml)
   + 1 teaspoons (5 ml) (the extra is to compensate for alcohol loss) of alcohol

   3000 x 20% THC = **600 mg THC**
   3000 x 5% CBD = **150 mg CBD**

   4 ounces (120 ml) of alcohol to fill 4, 1-ounce (30 ml) dropper bottles
   600 mg THC / 4 bottles = 150 mg THC per dropper bottle

150 mg CBD / 4 bottles = and 37.5 mg CBD per dropper bottle

With approximately 30 whole dropperful servings per bottle (1 ml of liquid serving at a time), the individual serving will be calculated as:
150 mg THC / 30 = 5 mg THC
37.5 mg CBD / 30 = 1.25 mg CBD

Similarly, if the milligrams of cannabinoids are already specified on the label as opposed to percentages, you can calculate straight from the label. **If you are using dried and/or cured homegrown flower that has not been tested, you can follow my method for testing the psychoactivity of the flower as described earlier in this chapter (page 142) to estimate serving sizes. This method is not suggested while you are still a novice. Always work with lab-tested cannabis plant material until you have gained more experience and understand your level of tolerance.**

2. Preheat the oven to 250°F (121°C). Place the pre-weighed flower into a covered baking dish and cover. Bake for 30 minutes, and remove from the oven and allow the flowers to cool.

3. Prepare a clean, glass canning jar. Add the decarboxylated cannabis flowers to the jar and crush/crumble them. Add the amount of alcohol necessary to fill the dropper bottles based on your calculations of how much cannabinoid per bottle and per serving you desire. Again, because these tinctures will result in a more intense 11 Hydroxy THC experience if the flowers you are using are rich in THCA, we go ahead and calculate based on the known percentages or milligrams without trying to calculate for loss. You can always adjust serving sizes after trying this tincture for the first time.

4. Allow these tinctures to extract for at least 2 weeks in a cool, dark cabinet. Shake frequently.

5. Decant the tincture and filter through cheesecloth into a large glass measuring cup. Using a funnel, fill the clean sanitized dropper bottles and affix the lids. Label each bottle with the total cannabinoid content and

6. Store in a cool, dark cabinet and **do not expose to light, heat, or air** in order to maintain the integrity of the cannabinoids. Use within 3 months for best results.

7. These tinctures may be used in either hot or cold beverages, on food, or taken directly from the bottle.

Beverage Emulsification Technique

I find that using acacia gum (sometimes known as acacia fiber), a culinary gum, is a pretty good way to emulsify cannabinoids in beverages whether I am using oil or an alcohol tincture. This is an easy product to find and is sold as a dietary fiber supplement. It will be a white powder that mixes readily with water.

Per 8 ounces (240 ml) of liquid, you will use 1 teaspoon (2.5 g) of acacia fiber powder. Add the powder to a cup or glass and the serving of cannabis tincture or oil. Add some of the beverage and whisk thoroughly. After whisking, add the rest of your beverage, whisk again, and enjoy.

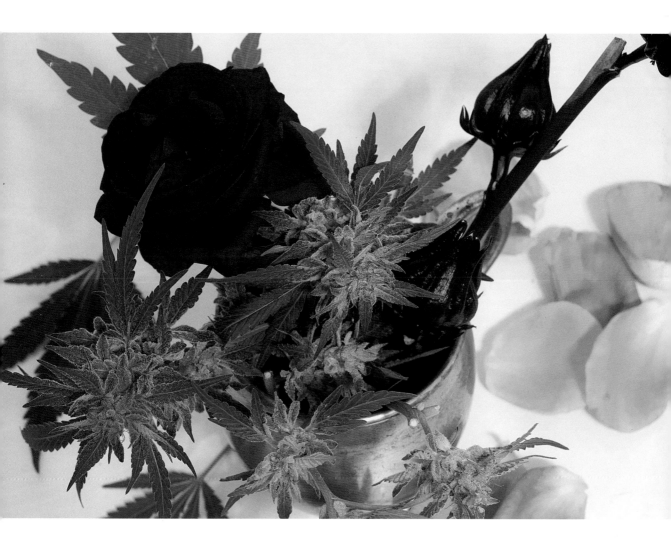

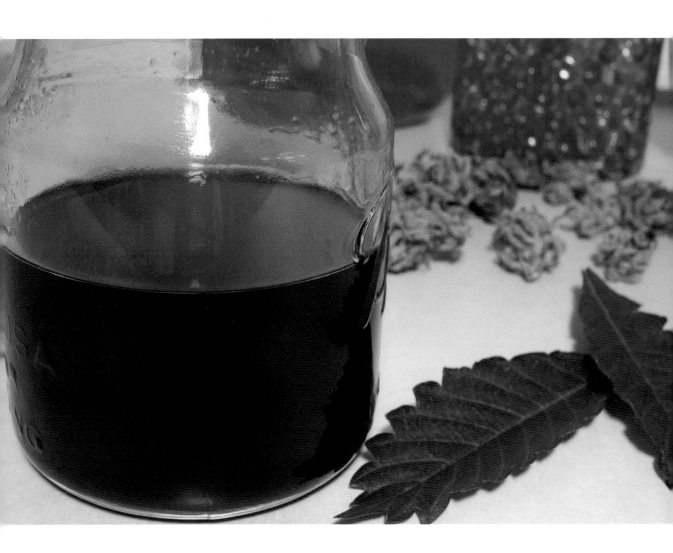

Oil Extractions

Cannabis oils are a convenient way to have cannabinoid on hand in serving sizes that are premeasured. You can take these oils directly, or add them to recipes or as toppings/ingredients for other foods like salad dressing or toast.

There are a few methods for making oils. The most convenient one for beginners that is also going to preserve a lot of the terpene content is a method I was taught by a farmer friend of mine who I have discussed in my other books. This is a slow cooker method that will process over a period of 24 hours on the lowest setting. But alas, there are faster methods, and I will cover that one, too, as it is similar to the tincturing method.

Before we choose either method, we need to do all of our calculations ahead of the recipe:

Calculate the total cannabinoid content of the raw cannabis flowers or hashish that you have purchased from the dispensary. If you have 2 grams of flower with 18% THC and 2% CBD, the calculation for total cannabinoids is as follows: 2 x 180 mg THC = **360 mg THC** and 2 x 20 mg CBD = **40 mg CBD.**

Next, calculate how much oil you would like to use. For our example, let's use 8 ounces (240 ml) of any oil or solid fat. There are 48 teaspoons (48 x 5 ml) in 8 ounces (240 ml), therefore each serving size of the oil or solid fat will be 1 teaspoon (5 ml), and each serving will contain **7.5 mg THC** and **0.83 mg CBD**. Milligrams of cannabinoid / number of servings = total cannabinoids for each serving.

Once you have weighed and measured the cannabis flower or hashish and the oils, and calculated the cannabinoid content for each serving size, write this down.

Slow Cooker Recipe

This recipe is intended for use with whole, dried cannabis flowers, as it will develop a flavor profile based on the flowers you use. Choose wisely! This is the best recipe to use with good-quality flower material, whereas the double-boiler method described next can be used with trim, lower-quality flower, or hashish and concentrates.

Instructions:

1. Set your slow cooker to the low setting. Add the cannabis flowers or hashish and fats/oils in the amount that you have calculated for your desired serving sizes of cannabinoids. Cover and keep covered. Stir only once or twice during the processing to retain terpene content.

2. Allow this to process on the low setting for at least 24 hours. My farmer friend has told me that this process has been carried out as long as 36 hours. The lower temperature processing for a longer period of time decarboxylates the cannabinoids using both time and temperature.

3. Turn off the slow cooker and allow this to stand covered until it is cool enough for you to handle. Filter the oil through cheesecloth and into a glass measuring cup. Squeeze out as much oil as possible from the plant material.

4. Check your written calculations to ensure that the amount of oil in the cup is equivalent to your calculation. If it is a little less, recalculate your serving size to match the amount of cannabinoid you desire in each serving.

5. Transfer to the bottle or jar where it will be stored. You may keep this in a cool, dark cabinet or in the refrigerator. Some oils will solidify in the refrigerator; keep this in mind when dispensing servings of the oil or fat. Label your container with total cannabinoid content, serving size content, and ingredients. Use within 3 months for best results.

You will need:
slow cooker
cannabis flowers
oil of your choice (I recommend MCT oil for this recipe)
cheesecloth
glass measuring cup
storage bottle or jar (amber glass is preferred)

Double Boiler Recipe

This recipe uses whole, dried, or cured cannabis flower products, trim, or hashish. Use this recipe, instead of the slow cooker recipe, if you would like to prepare cannabis infused butter or ghee.

Instructions:

You will need:
double boiler pan set
cannabis flowers, cannabis trim, hashish, or concentrates
fat or oil of your choice
cheesecloth
glass measuring cup
storage bottle or jar (amber glass is preferred)

1. Before beginning, prepare your calculations. These calculations will be the same as in the slow cooker recipe. Once you have written all of these down, weighed and measured both your cannabis plant material and your fats/oil, you are ready to begin.

2. Prepare a double boiler pan on the top of the stove. Add water to the bottom and add your cannabis material and oil/fat to the top pan. Set the heat to medium-low and cover.

3. When the water starts to simmer, uncover and stir the oil. Do this several times during the process. Watch the water pan to ensure it does not boil dry. Allow this to simmer for 60 to 90 minutes. A longer simmer time is suggested for higher elevations.

4. Remove from the stove and allow the oil to cool, covered, until you are able to handle it. Filter the oil through cheesecloth into a glass measuring cup. Squeeze out as much oil as possible from the plant material.

5. Check your written calculations to ensure that the amount of oil in the cup is equivalent to your calculation. If it is a little less, recalculate your serving size to match the amount of cannabinoid you desire in each serving.

6. Transfer to the bottle or jar where it will be stored. You may keep this in a cool, dark cabinet or in the refrigerator. Some oils will solidify in the refrigerator; keep this in mind when dispensing servings of the oil or fat. Label your container with total cannabinoid content, serving-size content, and ingredients. Use within 3 months for best results.

---

* If you are using dried and/or cured homegrown flower that has not been tested, you can follow my method of testing the psychoactivity of the flower as described earlier in this chapter (page 142) to calculate serving sizes. This method is not suggested while you are still a novice. Always work with lab-tested cannabis plant material until you have gained more experience and understand your level of tolerance.

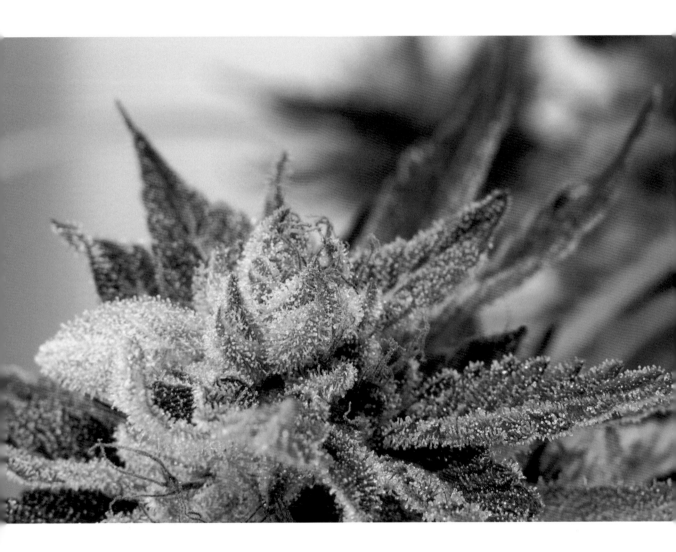

Cannabis Infusions with Other Medicinal and Culinary Herbs

In every book I have ever written, I place a lot of importance on learning to work with a variety of herbs, not just cannabis. Making a medicinal infusion is as easy as adding any of your favorite herbs and/or fruits during the processing of cannabis plant material in alcohol or oil and allowing the ingredients to infuse over a period of a few weeks. What is handy about doing infusions like this especially with fats and oils is that if no heat is applied you can create nonpsychoactive infusions.

Keep these tips handy if you would like to blend other herbs or fruit with your infusion:

- Only alcohol infusions containing 120- to 150-proof or higher alcohol will produce the best alcohol infusion of herbal blends. It's my opinion and I'm sticking with it. For example, if you want to make a cannabis tincture with fresh ginger slices and fresh, live, cannabis flowers, the higher proof will extract more compounds from the plant material and ensure shelf stability.
- **Alcohol infusions** like tinctures or tonics may use fresh, live plant material or dried plant material.
- **Oil infusions** like olive oil or MCT oil only use dried plant material, never fresh!

Using dried fruit or herbs is an excellent way to flavor extractions or to boost their effectiveness and serve as an entourage for the cannabinoids. Some recipe ideas for this are:

- Fresh turmeric slices, black peppercorns, and cannabis in an alcohol infusion as an anti-inflammatory herbal infusion
- Dried cherries, dried chamomile flowers, and cured cannabis in an alcohol infusion

- Fennel seed, dried orange peels, and cured cannabis in olive oil infusion for cold salad dressing
- Culinary oil infusion of cured cannabis, dried basil, dried oregano, sun-dried tomato, dried garlic, in olive oil.
- Culinary stir-fry oil consisting of avocado oil, sesame oil, dried Thai red peppers, cannabis, dried garlic, dried yuzu peels

The infusion process is simple: Just add all of your desired herbal and fruit ingredients to the desired alcohol or oil and allow these to infuse over a period of 2 to 4 weeks. Infusions may be formulated to create both psychoactive and nonpsychoactive finished products. **Remember: if an infusion, whether oil or alcohol, has heat applied (such as use as a cooking oil like in a stir-fry, or in a hot soup or beverage the cannabinoids in the infusion will decarboxylate and this may result in a psychoactive experience if you are using cannabis containing THC/THCV.** Always apply the methods of calculating cannabinoids as described in this chapter when adding cannabis to your herbal and fruit infusions.

Cooking with Cannabinoids: Recipe Ideas and Working Guide

I love good-quality boxed bakery mixes like brownie, cake, and cookies for the beginner. There are a lot of these to choose from, including brands that are sugar-free and gluten-free. These are helpful when you are first starting out making your own edibles because they require very little effort and give you the opportunity to focus on what is important as a beginner who has never made anything edible that contains cannabinoids—your oil and alcohol extractions or infusions and performing the proper calculations of cannabinoids.

Calculate and prepare your oil and butter extractions first, and then add these to the commercially prepared mixes of your choice. If desserts aren't your thing you can use your extractions in commercially prepared products like mac and cheese or pasta sauce. This is a great way to prepare accurate portioning of cannabinoids for the serving size you desire.

Single-serving beverages are another favorite for the beginner. This can be a cup of coffee or a glass of sparkling soda or anything else. Try one serving of cannabis-infused ghee or coconut oil in a cup of coffee for a supercharged bulletproof coffee! One serving of tincture in a cup of hot herbal tea as a night cap is amazing. Beverages are often faster onset than food, which can take up to 2 hours to affect you if it is psychoactive. Most of the time, beverages will take effect within 30 minutes in my experience.

Toast, bagels, and sandwiches are another way that you can use an oil extraction such as cannabis butter that you have prepared and portioned into serving sizes of cannabinoids that work best for you.

Salad dressings and sauces are the perfect medium for serving fats that have been infused with cannabinoids because they often contain herbs and other flavorful ingredients that contain aromatic terpenes which will enhance the entourage effect of your oil extraction.

Follow these steps for accurate portioning:

1. **Perform all calculations before beginning preparation.** Check your math at least twice. Know the exact dosage that you will be putting into each serving of food or beverage.
2. **Determine the exact number of servings you wish to create.** If you are using a commercially prepared boxed product, this does not have to to be the same number of servings on the label of the commercial boxed product. For example, a box of mac & cheese may specify that it has four servings. But, in practice, a box of mac & cheese ends up being one or two servings for one person. In this instance the amount of cannabis butter that you add will be a portion of cannabis butter equal to one or two servings of your desired dose of cannabinoids.
3. **Carefully portion the cannabis-infused oil or fat into a small dish or bowl away from your other ingredients until you are ready to add this to the recipe.** This will ensure that your cannabis oil extraction is not confused with any other ingredients and the exact dosage is accurate for the number of servings you want to create.
4. **Whenever possible, add your cannabis oil extraction as the very last ingredient.** This will also ensure that you have one last opportunity to check the portion size of the dosage you intend to create before adding it to your recipe.
5. **After your recipe is finished, carefully portion it out before consuming anything.** If this is a boxed brownie or cookie mix, portion it into the exact number of portions that you have calculated your desired individual doses for. If this is a sauce or salad dressing, portion out and measure each serving in a small spice bowl or other container instead of eyeballing a portion poured freely from the serving container directly on to food.

Proper Storage and Labeling of Cannabis Products

If you are going to have leftover portions, such as the case will be with a pan of brownies, for example, you will want to package and label these with care. The best place to keep your cannabis foods will be the refrigerator in closed containers which are clearly labeled with the date, contents, and dosage amount of each portion in the container. This goes for cannabis butter or other culinary oil extractions as well, and for these you will also want to add the dosage size in addition to the other information on the label. I cannot stress how critical this is because these products are an accident waiting to happen if they are not stored and labeled correctly. **There is one additional step if there are children or others in the home who need supervision like an elderly person with dementia: Use a locking container for all cannabis preparations and cannabis products whether or not the products are in the refrigerator.**

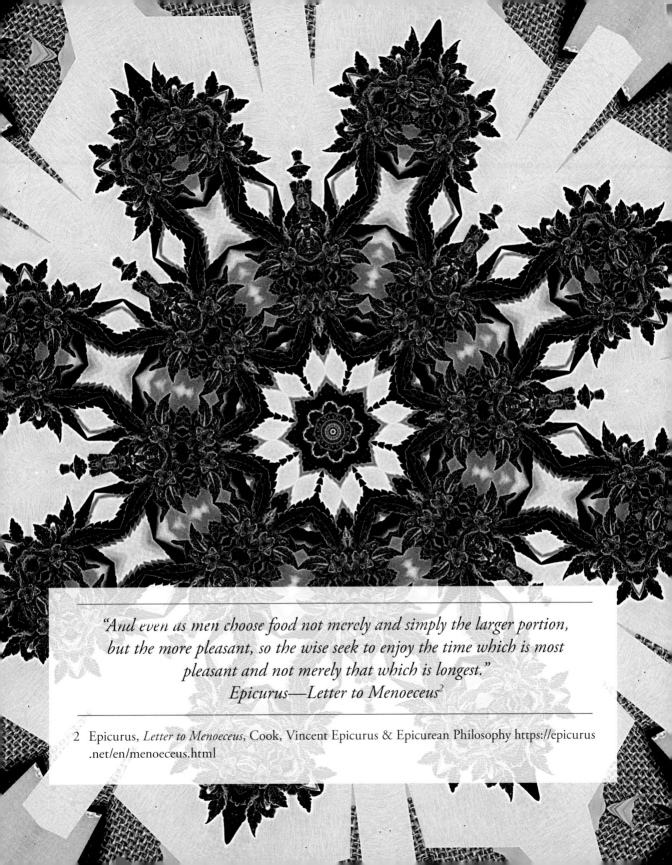

"And even as men choose food not merely and simply the larger portion, but the more pleasant, so the wise seek to enjoy the time which is most pleasant and not merely that which is longest."
Epicurus—Letter to Menoeceus[2]

2 Epicurus, *Letter to Menoeceus*, Cook, Vincent Epicurus & Epicurean Philosophy https://epicurus .net/en/menoeceus.html

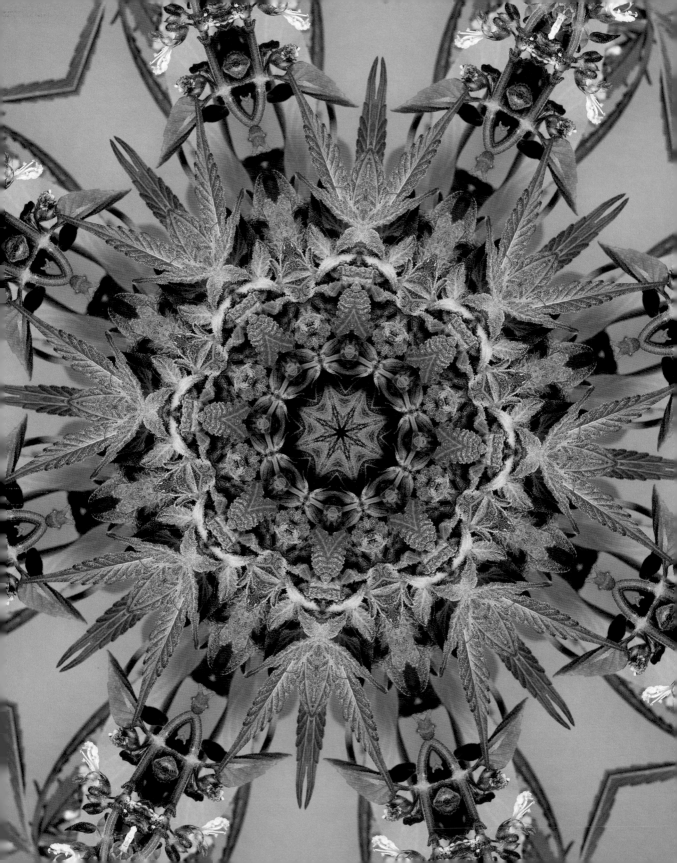

RESOURCES

Some ingredients and tools mentioned in this book may not be readily available at a local shop. For these less-common ingredients and tools, these are my most recommended resources based on personal experience with the quality and pricing that are offered for.

Amazon: I recommend them in many of my books because it's the biggest marketplace and carries many hard-to-find items. https://www.amazon.com

Mountain Rose Herbs: This is a reliable herbal shop that sells many fine raw herbal ingredients https://mountainroseherbs.com/

Greenpoint Seeds: A mail-order cannabis seed bank in the United States offering a wide selection of feminized seeds to get you started, both CBD and regular seeds https://green pointseeds.com/

Master Grower and Artisan List

This book covers a very basic overview of topics like growing and hash making for beginners. If these topics interest you, I suggest that you check out these masters of the craft to learn more.

Frenchy Cannoli: A true master of the art of traditional hashish-making, learning from Frenchy is essential if you are growing your own cannabis and want to try your hand at traditional hashish craft. Unfortunately, Frenchy is no longer with us in this universe, but his work and free classes in traditional hashish making live on. https://www.youtube.com/c /FrenchyCannoli | https://frenchycannoli.com/

Donnie Danko: A master of the grow, Donnie has great resources for beginners who would like to stretch their wings and take growing to another level. Check out his podcast and book for beginners just like you! https://podcasts.apple.com/us/podcast/grow-bud-yourself/ id453789227 | https://amzn.to/3H9DHR9

Safeeakh: My friend operates Safeeakh Farms and is a master grower of many interesting and rare cannabis phenotypes and strains. His work is the "next-level" of everything cannabis. https://safeeakh.org/

Jorge Cervantes: Jorge is certainly a heavyweight in the area of cannabis cultivation and has written very comprehensive texts on the subject. I recommend these for a real deep dive into growing. https://amzn.to/33CLB7J | https://www.youtube.com/c/jorgecervantesmj

Bonni Goldstein, MD: Dr. Goldstein is a doctor who understands why you want to use cannabis and wants to help you with evidence- and science-based approaches. This is the book to take with you to your doctor's office for those who have skeptical doctors! https://amzn.to/3sUEVdT

CONVERSION CHART

Metric and Imperial Conversions

(These conversions are rounded for convenience)

Ingredient	Cups/ Tablespoons/ Teaspoons	Ounces	Grams/ Milliliters
Fruit, dried	1 cup	4 ounces	120 grams
Fruits or veggies, chopped	1 cup	5 to 7 ounces	145 to 200 grams
Fruits or veggies, puréed	1 cup	8.5 ounces	245 grams
Honey, maple syrup, or corn syrup	1 tablespoon	0.75 ounce	20 grams (15 milliliters)
Liquids: cream, milk, water, or juice	1 cup	8 fluid ounces	240 milliliters
Salt	1 teaspoon	0.2 ounces	6 grams
Spices: cinnamon, cloves, ginger, or nutmeg (ground)	1 teaspoon	0.2 ounce	2.5–3 grams
Sugar, brown, firmly packed	1 cup	8 ounces	200 grams
Sugar, white	1 cup/ 1 tablespoon	8 ounces/ 0.5 ounce	200 grams/ 12.5 grams
Vanilla extract	1 teaspoon	0.2 ounce	5 milliliters

Liquids

8 fluid ounces = 1 cup = ½ pint
16 fluid ounces = 2 cups = 1 pint
32 fluid ounces = 4 cups = 1 quart
128 fluid ounces = 16 cups = 1 gallon

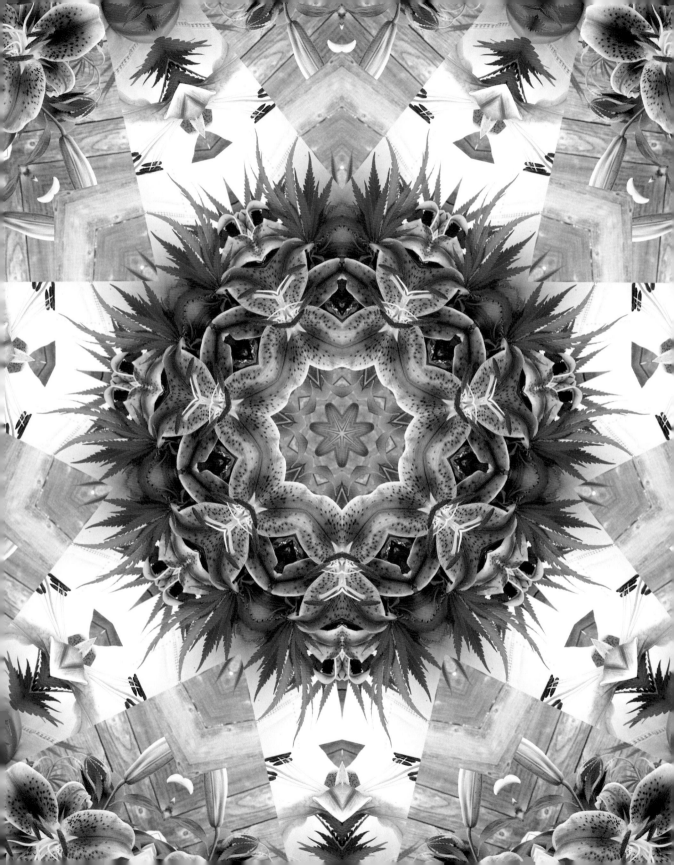

INDEX

mental illness, 82–83
mid-shelf flower, 90–91
mindfulness, 69–73
miso soup, 65
molasses, 51, 57

N

Naoko's Japanese Cannabis Leaf Condiment, 63
nuts, 97

O

odor, 40–41, 76
oil
    in extraction, 140
    extractions, 149–151
    full-extract cannabis, 92
    infusions, 153
O'Shaughnessy, William, 7–8

P

Persia, 3
pills, 99
pipe, fruit, 77–78
pizza, 97
plant
    from feminized seed *vs.* clone, 53–55
    first, 48–60
    grow setup for single, 51–53
    harvesting, 59–60
    pot for, 55
    watering, 55–56, 57
plant products, cannabis, 43–48
pollen, 45
pot (container), 55
prepared meal, 97
pre-rolls, 95
prohibition, 11–20

R

radicle, 24
recipes
    nonpsychoactive, 61–65
    topical/spa products, 118–136
roll-ons, 120–121
root cap, 24
roots, 45
rootworking salve, 129–130
rosin, 46, 92–93
RSO, 92
rubs, 101, 116, 131–133

S

safety, 80
Sajous, Charles, 13
salad dressing, 155
salves, 101, 116, 118–119, 123–124, 129–130
sandwiches, 155
sanitary practices, 107
sativa strains, 47
sauces, 155
scissors, 51–52
Scythians, 2, 3
seed, 24, 44
seed coat, 24
seedling, 24
Seneca, 67
shatter, 94
shoot apex, 24
shrines, 5–6
skincare products, 101–102
slow cooker extraction, 150
smoking, in first experience, 81–82
snacks, 71, 97
soil, 51, 56